HEALTHCARE HEROES

THE MEDICAL CAREERS GUIDE

Mary Choy
PharmD, BCGP, FASHP

Michele B. Kaufman
PharmD, BCGP

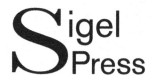

Healthcare Heroes: The Medical Careers Guide

ISBN: 978-1-905941-31-5

Sigel Press
4403 Belmont Court
Medina, Ohio 44256

Visit us at www.sigelpress.com

Cover and internal design by Harp Mando

Printed in the United States of America.
Printed on 100% recycled, 100% post-consumer waste paper.

MBK - To my parents, Elaine and Harold Kaufman, whose lives were dedicated to education and helping others, and to my spouse, Jo Ellen for believing in me and this book.

* * *

MC - To my mother, the strongest woman I know — who inspired me to follow my dreams and find my passion in pharmacy. To my high school sweetheart and husband, Eric, and my children — Elise and Ethan, you are my world.

Contents

Preface

We were interested in science at an early age and knew that science would play a big part in our careers. As pharmacists passionate about pharmacy and healthcare, friends and family often ask us for guidance on careers. Some of the comments or questions people have asked us are, "I'm interested in a career in healthcare, but I don't know what I should do," or "Can you tell me more about pharmacy and other professions?" Both parents and their children who were at a crossroads of choosing careers made such comments and asked these questions. Finding a satisfying career is an important stage in life and good guidance is the key to success. Finding the right career is an investment in yourself. We were lucky to find the careers that we enjoy and are right for us. We never think of our work as just a job... we are *always* passionate about challenging ourselves every day and motivating others to achieve their potential.

If you've picked up this book, you are most likely at a crossroads of choosing your career, or perhaps you are helping a friend or family member to delve deeper into researching a particular career. Your initial thought might be, "Why would pharmacists write a career book?" We took the "Oath of a Pharmacist" upon graduating from pharmacy school. The American Pharmacists Association developed this oath and other professional pharmacy associations and colleges of pharmacy have adopted this as a code of ethics. In this oath, in addition to optimizing patient care, the statement that stands out most to us is: "I will utilize my knowledge, skills, experiences and values to prepare the next generation of pharmacists." Throughout our careers, we have followed this oath and mentored numerous students in the medical field to conduct research, give presentations, publish articles and teach others, in order to optimize their career. In today's marketplace, competitive advantage is invaluable, and it begins with knowledge. We have found it especially rewarding to see our students become successful practitioners and find fulfillment and personal success in their careers. We know that not everyone has a mentor readily available for guidance. We hope this book will help many individuals find their inspiration and trust that it will serve as a blueprint for finding a successful career.

We strive to bring real value to our readers and wanted to share the experiences of these healthcare professionals to inspire everyone to find the career that is right for them. When we speak about our careers — whether it's one-to-one or on the auditorium stage — we personalize our experiences for our audience. Although we have taught and mentored numerous students interested in pursuing a healthcare career, we saw that our impact was still minimal. Many individuals still had unanswered career questions. Hence, came our idea for the book...how can we help young adults interested in understanding about healthcare learn about the many different careers? Why wait for the next career day to learn about the various professions when these individuals can read about the different professions in advance? Readers can also use this book as a resource to develop their questions, and bring them to the next career fair. Personalization is very important to us and our concept was to spotlight each healthcare professional, for our readers to experience the "personal touch." We developed a way to personalize each healthcare provider career and considered that our readers would appreciate a new information format, as these healthcare experts describe their professions and provide in-depth information for readers. It was interesting for us to read the life experiences of how our contributors, experts in their field, became who they are today and we hope you, our readers, agree.

We knew we were on the right path when we received poignant feedback from our young adult peer reviewers, ages 11-18 years. Here are a few of the comments that truly resonated with us: *"A genuine lifesaver filled with chapters of professionals telling you everything you need to know about their job, it was written in a way that was fun to read,"* *"It gives the reader a real sense of the business."* Another comment was: *"If you know you want to be a healthcare professional, whether it's in the emergency room or in the laboratory, then this book is right for you. If you don't know at all if you want to be a healthcare professional, then this book is STILL right for you."*

Readers are encouraged to explore and learn about different careers beginning in elementary school. These days, it is the norm for schools to hold career days, where parents are welcomed into the school to speak to the different grades about their careers. We have even seen these career day events done as early as kindergarten! Even though there are over a hundred types of healthcare professions, and thousands of healthcare professionals, most people are not familiar with the diverse career opportunities and areas of practice available within the health field. Adults, much less young adults, often do not have exposure to a vast variety of healthcare professionals, except perhaps a physician, a dentist, a nurse, a pharmacist and maybe a dental hygienist. Through our market research, we discovered that our concept was unique and that there is a need for a resource that will equip readers with the knowledge necessary to guide their healthcare career path.

We hope that you find this book fun to read, and that it will be a useful resource and guide for readers of all ages, whether they are in middle school, high school, college or already out in the workforce. Our contributors are healthcare professionals who are ambitious, resourceful, innovative, adaptive — and renowned forces of change — from clinicians to technologists. They work in hospitals, offices, clinics, laboratories and in the field. They are recognized locally, regionally, and nationally for their accomplishments and expertise. Our goal was to have them share their extensive knowledge as part of their journey into each of their professions. We hope this insightful information can also help our adult readers who are interested in a career change to a healthcare profession.

This book is your career guide, showing you the requirements and core strategies to become a healthcare professional. From concept to writing, this book has been our passion project for the past several years. We hope you enjoy reading it as much as we have enjoyed writing it.

Acknowledgements

We are grateful to all the wonderful people in our lives who inspired us along the way to create this resource that will hopefully serve as a helpful guide for readers on finding their career paths. We had so much fun writing this book and we are thankful for our family and friends who responded to our late-night texts and phone calls — it was truly a community effort. We knew our adult peer reviewers would provide honest reviews of the book — and they did! Special thanks to Christina Law for her candid opinions. In one of our brainstorming sessions, we took it a step further and thought it would be a fantastic idea to have young adults serve as peer reviewers and get a first look at the book. We are so proud of these young adults (ages 11-18) who provided their thoughtful comments and valuable insight: Sean Feeney, Christopher Liantonio, Gianna Micelli, William Nasella, Keane Robinson, Sage Robinson, Tess Robinson, Isabella Stelter and Joey Yu.

As coauthors working together for extended periods of time on projects throughout the years, we have much in common with each other (besides our passion for pharmacy). First, our names both start with an M and we love our brothers and want to thank them for always being there for us. To Raymond Choy, for being a great brother to Mary, supplying her with endless food deliveries (food is somehow always en route during the writing sessions), being the best uncle to the kids and providing unfiltered thoughts on the book. To Roy S. Kaufman, for being a great brother to Michele, always looking out for the best interest of this book, and for your direction in navigating the publishing process and the legal aspects of publishing. Thank you both!

Finally, we would like to thank our contributors for sharing their expertise with us. We would like to thank Deborah Frank, NP, for her input to the nursing profession chapter. Also, we give a big shout-out to Suzanne Fiore Photography for the photo session.

Many thanks to our publisher, Sigel Press — we are so lucky to have the dream team as our partners in this project.

About the Editors

Mary Choy, PharmD, BCGP, FASHP, has over 15 years of pharmacy practice, public health and higher education experience. She currently serves as the President of EMCY Medical Communications in New York City. Her focus is on brand strategy and healthcare communications. She is also the Director of Pharmacy Practice for the New York State Council of Health-System Pharmacists.

Mary graduated with honors and received a Doctor of Pharmacy degree from St. John's University. She then completed a residency at the Veteran Affairs New York Harbor Healthcare System, where she provided care for the veterans who served our country. She is board certified in geriatric pharmacotherapy. As a practicing pharmacist, Mary has experience within the community, academic, hospital, and pharmaceutical industry settings. As founding faculty and a pharmacy professor at Touro College of Pharmacy, she developed an internal medicine/geriatrics clinical practice site and served as a clinical pharmacist at Metropolitan Hospital, both of which are in Harlem. Prior to this appointment, she was a pharmacy professor at St. John's University and was a nephrology/transplant clinical pharmacist at Northwell Health North Shore University Hospital in Manhasset. Mary is published in the medical literature and is frequently invited to speak at professional conferences. She has published her research on clinical findings, assessment and public health in various scholarly journals. She particularly enjoys speaking at platforms highlighting careers in healthcare, as well as providing mentorship and guidance to students on their research and career goals.

Mary is an exemplary leader with a passion for advancing healthcare, education and service to the community. She is an active member and leader in professional organizations at both the state and national level. She has held multiple leadership roles, including serving as President of the New York City Society of Health-System Pharmacists (NYCSHP). She has also served on numerous state and national boards and advisory councils. Her leadership and devotion to public health and the pharmacy profession are exemplified through her work promoting public health awareness related to smoking cessation, improving low immunization rates and improving diabetes management and other health conditions that minorities face in the New York City area. She has partnered with several groups (including the New York City Department of Health & Mental Hygiene, the New York University Center for the Study of Asian American Health, the New York City Coalition for a Smoke-Free City, the Brooklyn Smoke-Free Partnership and the Chinese-American Planning Council) to train community health workers, conduct health fairs and provide immunizations. She is well recognized by the profession and community for her efforts in leadership and research, and has appeared on the NBC Today Show, SinoVision TV and has been featured in newspapers and magazines. She is a Fellow of the American Society of Health-System Pharmacists (ASHP), as well as a recipient of several prestigious honors, including the ASHP-ABHP Joint Leadership Award, American Pharmacists Association Immunization Champion Award, New York City Council Citation, New York State Assembly Citation and the NYCSHP Harold Neham Award.

Michele B. Kaufman, PharmD, BCGP, has over 30 years of pharmacy practice, medical writing and higher education experience. She is currently a Pharmacist at NewYork-Presbyterian Hospital - Lower Manhattan and a medical writer and editor for medical and pharmacy journals. Michele received her Bachelor of Science in Pharmacy from the University of Rhode Island (URI) College of Pharmacy, and her Doctor of Pharmacy degree from Massachusetts College of Pharmacy and Allied Health Sciences in Boston, MA. Michele also completed a Drug Information Fellowship at the URI Drug Information Center/Roger Williams Medical Center in Providence, RI. She is a registered pharmacist and a Board Certified Geriatric Pharmacist (BCGP).

As a practicing pharmacist, Michele has experience within the community, in the pharmaceutical industry as a product development pharmacist/scientist, as a poison information specialist, as a clinical assistant professor of pharmacy at St. John's University, as a drug information specialist, as a geriatric pharmacy project leader/pharmacy case manager in managed care pharmacy, as a clinical pharmacist in managed care and in a hospital, as a pharmacy college experiential preceptor and as a medical education writer and director of quality. While a product development pharmacist in the pharmaceutical industry, Michele was a co-inventor of Pineapple-flavored Colyte® and Colyte® Flavor Packs, with patents issued. In addition, Michele enjoys mentoring students on pharmacy, writing and potential career paths. She has published many peer-reviewed and other medically oriented articles throughout her career, and has lectured on pharmacy and health-related topics. Michele is an active member of numerous professional societies for healthcare providers, pharmacists and writers, and has served on the board of many organizations. She is a member of the editorial board for the *Pharmacy & Therapeutics (P&T) Journal*. She created and manages the Pharmacovigilance Forum for *P&T Journal*. She is also a writer for the "Drug Updates" column for *The Rheumatologist*. She serves as a member of the Callen-Lorde Community Health Center's Clinical Care Committee in New York City. Michele is the recipient of two prestigious awards from the NYCSHP, the Harold Neham Award and the Joel Yellin Award. She is also a past recipient (2015) of the Excellence in Pharmacy Employee of the Year Award from the Pharmacy Department at NewYork-Presbyterian Hospital - Lower Manhattan and the Academy of Managed Care Pharmacy Individual Contributor Award (2013).

Contributors

Richard C. Adrian, BA

Rich was raised on Long Island, New York, and received his BA degree in Business Administration from Providence College in 1993. He is currently an Executive Sales Representative for Janssen Pharmaceuticals in New York, New York. Rich has experience selling pharmaceuticals in the following areas: Anti-Infectives, Cardiovascular/Metabolic, Pain Management, Urology, and Biologics. He currently sells Janssen's Cardiovascular and Metabolism portfolio to hospitals in Lower Manhattan, New York City. He has won many company awards throughout his career including: District Sales Representative of the Year, Regional Representative of the Year, and was most recently recognized as a top sales representative nationwide by winning the President's Circle Award at Janssen Pharmaceuticals in 2015, 2016 and 2017. He enjoys cooking, traveling and golf.

Paul S. Albicocco, DMD, MS

Paul received a BS degree in Biology at Wagner College on Staten Island and then completed an MS in Microbiology/Bacteriology (also at Wagner College). He then received his DMD from Rutgers School of Dental Medicine. He completed a post-graduate residency program at Maimonides Medical Center in Brooklyn, New York. Since completing his training, he owns and runs a private dental practice in Staten Island, New York. As a member of the American Dental Association he has served many roles including past president of the Richmond Country Dental Society and is the current Vice President of the Second District Dental Society of New York. While serving on the New York State Dental Association (NYSDA) Council for Dental Licensure and as past chairperson of the Council on Dental Practice for New York State, he has assisted in passing legislation helping dentists and patients in New York State in advancing dental care. He has lectured on topics such as oral cancer detection, child abuse and reporting, and forensic dental identification. He continues to educate practicing dentists and dental hygienists in the community. During the recovery efforts of September 11, 2001, he became a member of the forensic dental identification unit tasked in identifying the remains of victims through dental records. He continues to serve as a member of the forensic identification unit in the event of a natural or manmade disaster, if human remains need identification. Paul enjoys traveling with his family and learning about the many different cultures and traditions of people around the world. Having been a Boy Scout and achieving the rank of Eagle Scout, he still enjoys camping and outdoor activities with his family. For more information visit: http://www.dralbicocco.com/.

Suzannah Callaghan, LCSW-R

Suzannah grew up in Atlanta, Georgia. She received her BA in Psychology and Women's Studies from Swarthmore College in Pennsylvania and completed her MS in Social Work at Columbia University in 2002. She has worked in areas of social work including domestic violence, sexual assault and issues related to aging. After this, she decided to shift her focus, and work with mentally ill adults in both the hospital inpatient psychiatric unit setting, as well as in the outpatient psychiatric settings. She spent seven years offering mental health treatment in a university and founding the first Counseling Centers at Touro College of Osteopathic Medicine and at Touro College of Pharmacy. After her time working in higher education, she returned to working in the setting that she loves most, the outpatient psychiatric hospital setting. In this setting she offers therapy to adults with severe and persistent mental illness as a social worker at a state psychiatric hospital. She also has a private adult therapy practice in Brooklyn. Her clinical focus is Gestalt Therapy, a therapeutic approach that deeply focuses on the therapeutic relationship as a tool for understanding how the client/patient interacts with his or her world. Additionally, she has completed certifications in trauma work, somatic psychotherapy, sex therapy, dream analysis and dialectical behavioral therapy. When not working as a therapist, Suzannah loves gardening, crocheting, communing with nature, reading novels and horsing around with her energetic and playful twins.

Young-Ju Chang, BS, R.T.(R)(MR) ARRT, CRT

Young-Ju went to school in the military as a radiology technologist. She then received a BS in Healthcare Management, with an emphasis in Radiologic Science from Oregon Institute of Technology, Klamath Falls, Oregon. She is currently a pediatric magnetic resonance imaging (MRI) technologist at Lucile Packard Children's Hospital in Palo Alto, California. She has been imaging patients since 2003, using different imaging equipment, such as radiography, fluoroscopy, portable X-ray machines, mammography, computed tomography and high field MRI scanners. She is nationally certified with the American Registry of Radiologic Technologists in both Radiography and Magnetic Resonance Imaging and licensed with California as a Radiology Technologist. She is a member of the Society of Magnetic Resonance Technologists.

Randal Chinnock, BS

Randal received his BS in Engineering Physics from the University of Colorado, and studied Mechanics and Materials Science at Johns Hopkins University. He is a biomedical engineer and serial entrepreneur. He has founded four companies involved in optical and medical devices. Most recently, he founded and directs the Southbridge Tech Incubator (STI). STI is a privately held collaborative workspace aimed to provide an environment where startup companies can create, build, interact, and share ideas and resources. A wide variety of mentors, advisors, consultants and suppliers are available to help tenants' teams deal with the Food and Drug Administration (FDA), meet their product development goals and achieve commercial success.

Randal is also the Founder and Chief Executive Officer (CEO) of Optimum Technologies, Inc (OTI). Since its founding in 1994, the firm has focused on helping clients commercialize technologies that use light to diagnose and treat disease. The OTI team has contributed to the successful launch of scores of medical devices and laboratory instruments based on optical technologies. Areas of expertise include ophthalmic instruments, disposable endoscopic cameras, vision systems for surgical robots, 3D vision systems, retinal imaging, spectroscopy, laser delivery systems and optical cancer detection. Randal's 40 years of experience include positions in engineering, manufacturing, marketing and general management at several companies engaged in electro-optical devices and systems. Randal is also a mentor to entrepreneurs, a judge of senior biomedical engineering projects at two universities, an advisor to startup companies and a STEM evangelist who introduces the field of biomedical engineering to primary and secondary school students. In his free time, he likes to build things, swim, cook, sing in a chorus and watch movies - preferably with his wife and two grown children. He lives in Northeastern Connecticut and New York City. For more information visit: https://southbridgetechincubator. com/ and https://www.optimum-tech.com/.

Kamilla Danilova, DPM

Kamilla immigrated to the United States at the age of 16 from Baku, Azerbaijan, which was part of the former Soviet Union. Her family settled in Brooklyn, New York, where she attended Franklin Delano Roosevelt High School for a year and a half. She then received a BA in Psychology at Hunter College, City University of New York, in a pre-medicine/pre-dental program. She switched from her pre-dental program to podiatry and graduated from the New York School of Podiatric Medicine (NYCPM). She completed a three-year surgical residency at Mount Sinai Beth Israel Medical Center, New York City, and works as a private practice podiatrist in New York City. She enjoys spending time with her husband and children. For more information visit: http://www.tdpodiatry.com/.

Eileen DeVries, BSN, RN, OCN, CBCN

Eileen received her diploma in Nursing at Pilgrim State Psychiatric Center. She had many varied jobs in the nursing field including Cardiac Intensive Care Unit (ICU), Medical/Surgical nursing, Intravenous (IV) Team Manager and IV Home Care, during the height of the AIDS epidemic. Eileen has worked in the field of Oncology for the last 20 years. After working as a nurse for 33 years, Eileen returned to school and earned her BSN. She holds certifications in Oncology Nursing (OCN) and Breast Cancer (CBCN). Eileen has also been a past president and founding member of the Intravenous Nursing Society, Long Island chapter, and continues to participate in the Oncology Nursing Society, New York City chapter. She has lectured to nurses and patients in many settings including to patient support groups and at conferences. She currently works in an outpatient Oncology practice affiliated with a hospital and is Unit Council President for the outpatient departments of her hospital. She enjoys traveling and meeting new people.

Carolyn DiMicco, MBA, RD, CDN, CNSC

Carolyn is a Registered Dietitian with over seven years' experience ranging from critical care nutrition to long-term care and hospice. Carolyn has a passion for pediatric nutrition care, and is committed to providing person-centered, trauma-informed care to the children that she serves. She is currently working as a Quality Systems Analyst for Elizabeth Seton Pediatric Center in Yonkers, New York– a pediatric long-term care center for medically fragile children ages birth to 21 years old. Carolyn is passionate about improving access to healthcare for those in need. A Westchester, New York native, Carolyn is well-versed in the diverse nutrition and health needs across the state and strives to advocate for her patients to overcome social determinants of health. Carolyn holds a BS in Nutrition and Dietetics from the University of Rhode Island, and an MBA in Healthcare Administration from the City University of New York (CUNY) Baruch College. Carolyn enjoys public speaking engagements at nutrition conferences, such as the New York State Women Infants and Children (WIC) Association Conference.

Mark Fusco, CST

Mark attended St. Johns University and CUNY in New York, studying Psychology and Spanish. He was a New York State Emergency Medical Technician (EMT) scoring 100% on the state exam. At that time, no one had achieved that score in six years. He also attended the French Culinary Institute in New York City where he received a Grande Diplome in Culinary Arts. Most recently he attended the Staten Island University Hospital Surgical Technician Training Program obtaining his Certification in Surgical Technology. He is currently employed as a Certified Surgical Technician at Staten Island University Hospital, a member of Northwell Health, New York. Mark's greatest personal satisfactions include (1) involvement with a surgical team during a femur fracture repair, performing cardiopulmonary resuscitation (CPR) on a patient that had "coded" during surgery (lost their heartbeat), and (2) the ability to help give patients back to their family following surgery.

Pamela J. Ginsberg, PhD

Pamela is a licensed psychologist in private practice in Doylestown, Pennsylvania. She specializes in women's health and psycho-oncology. She is on the Board of Directors for the Cancer Support Community of Greater Philadelphia, the Medical Advisory Board for KNOWoncology, which is the research database for the Oncology Association of Naturopathic Physicians and on the medical staff at Doylestown Hospital. Dr. Ginsberg received her Ph.D. in Counseling Psychology at Ball State University in 1993 and completed her doctoral internship at the Berkshire Medical Center in Pittsfield, Massachusetts, where she was involved in integrating family systems treatment and medical illness. She is a consultant and speaker for several local and national cancer support organizations, including Living Beyond Breast Cancer, Unite for Her and The Healing Consciousness Foundation. She is the chair of the medical advisory board for the Cancer Support Community of Greater Philadelphia, and the co-chair of the Health and Wellness committee of the Central Bucks County Chamber of Commerce. She is a member of the American Psycho-Social Oncology Society, the American Psychological Association, the Society of Health Psychology and a fellow of the Pennsylvania Psychological Association. Visit https://www.pginsbergphd.com/ to learn more about her practice.

Michael Greco, PhD, DNP, CRNA

Michael is an Assistant Professor of Nursing at Hofstra University in the Graduate School of Nursing and in the Physician Assistant Studies. He also serves as the Director of Nurse Anesthesia Services for Northwell Health in New York. Michael presently oversees the Certified Registered Nurse Anesthetist (CRNA) practice at seven medical centers throughout the New York area. Michael received his Ph.D. in Philosophy from Barry University in Miami Shores, Florida, his Doctorate in Nursing Practice (DNP) from the University of Alabama and his MS in Nurse Anesthesia from the State University of New York (SUNY) Downstate, Brooklyn, New York and his BS in nursing education from Niagara University, Buffalo, New York. Michael is the Chair of the National Professional Development Committee for the American Association of Nurse Anesthetists. He shares his passion for the science of anesthesia and peri-anesthesia care all over the country through lecturing. In addition, he has disseminated his knowledge as an author of numerous publications. Michael recently stepped down as the Program Director of the CRNA program at Columbia University and is in the process of writing the CRNA curriculum for Hofstra University in New York to open their first school on Long Island. Michael has a global footprint and has volunteered in numerous South American Countries as a CRNA during surgical missions.

Zachary Green, BA

Zachary has been a Pharmacy Technician Certification Board (PTCB) certified technician since 2008. He currently serves as the Associate Director of Partnership Development at PTCB. In this role, he manages educator and employer advocate program accounts. He also assists with the various activities surrounding PTCB's stakeholder relationships working with national and state pharmacy associations and state boards of pharmacy. Prior to joining PTCB, Zachary worked in the field as a Pharmacy Technician at Mount Carmel West Hospital in Columbus, Ohio. He earned his BA in Public Affairs, with research distinction, and a minor in Public Health at The Ohio State University. His study of Public Affairs focused specifically on pharmacy policy analysis where he researched surrounding policies dealing with pharmaceutical waste.

Julie Gruber, PA-C, MPAS

Julie is a graduate of the Touro College School of Health Sciences Physician Assistant Program. She currently is a Manager of Advanced Practice Providers (Physician Assistants [PAs] and Nurse Practitioners [NPs]) in the Urgent Care and Clinical Decision Unit at Memorial Sloan Kettering Cancer Center in New York City. Previously she was a Senior PA at New York-Presbyterian Hospital for over five years. In 2016, she was awarded the New York Presbyterian - Physician Assistant of the Year, for which she is very proud. Her greatest accomplishment was becoming a PA and working in critical care settings alongside other amazing providers.

Michael Lazara, DPT

Mike grew up in Syracuse, New York, and graduated from Stony Brook University in 2015 with a Doctorate of Physical Therapy degree. For three years after graduating, he worked as a physical therapist in New York City. Subsequently he has been working as the clinic manager for a private outpatient orthopedic company in Florida. As an orthopedic physical therapist, he treats a variety of musculoskeletal conditions including patients who have undergone total knee and hip replacements, rotator cuff repairs, athletic shoulder and hip injuries and patients with lower back and neck pain. He is also an American Physical Therapy Association Credentialed Clinical Instructor and has had the opportunity to attend several continuing education courses with a primary focus on evaluation and treatment of the shoulder and cervical spine, as well as courses on functional rehabilitation and orthopedic manual therapy techniques. He is a huge fan of the Syracuse Orange football and basketball teams. His hobbies include playing basketball and hiking.

Rova Lee-Huang, MS, CLT

Rova attended New York University for her undergraduate studies. She received her BA in Biology and then completed an MS degree at Long Island University in Pharmacology. At that time the medical technology field did not require licensing and only required a bachelor's degree. She started her medical laboratory career in the Department of Mycology at Bellevue Hospital in New York City. After a year, she moved into a position that required more experience, working in Microbiology at the Veterans Administration Medical Center in Manhattan and Brooklyn, New York. When licensing became a requirement, she obtained a New York State Clinical Laboratory Technologist license to continue her career in the clinical laboratory. During her time as a microbiology laboratory technologist, she helped develop a Molecular Microbiology section. It was in that time that she realized her expertise was in molecular biology. Soon she moved into a Molecular Pathology laboratory at Northwell Laboratories, part of North Shore University Hospital in Manhasset, New York, that specialized in performing highly complex genetic testing. After working as a molecular pathology technologist for two years she was promoted to technical specialist and subsequently to lead technologist. Currently she trains new laboratory technologists in performing molecular tests such as real time polymerase chain reactions (PCR) to perform molecular testing for cancer patients.

Anne Llewellyn, RN-C, MS, BHSA, CRRN

Anne received her BA from Barry University in Florida and her MA from the University of St. Francis in Pennsylvania. She obtained her nursing degree at Hahnemann University in Philadelphia. She is an independent Nurse Case Manager, working for herself. Her role is mostly as an educator and a mentor to nurses and other professionals who go into case management/ care coordination. She holds national certifications in case management and rehabilitation. Her most impressive accomplishment has been working as a nurse. Nursing has opened doors to various jobs and roles that have enhanced her personally and professionally. She feels that she has been incredibly lucky as a nurse with over 40 years of experience in many different areas of the healthcare system. In 2015, she received the "Lifetime Achievement Award" from the Case Management Society of America (CMSA). The award meant a great deal to her and she was humbled to accept the award in front of family, friends and colleagues at the 2015 CMSA Annual Conference. She belongs to an International Service Organization that provides service projects in the community for the deaf and hard of hearing and women and disadvantaged children. It has been a great way for her to give back to her community and to people in need. Anne also serves on her local case management chapter board and does her best to be an ambassador for the profession of nursing and case management. Since 1988, she has lived in Fort Lauderdale, Florida, with her husband. She loves the Fort Lauderdale lifestyle, the water, the weather and the ability to swim and fish year-round. For more information visit: https://www. linkedin.com/in/allewellyn/.

Catherine Monchik, BA, RDH

Catherine Monchik is a registered dental hygienist. She graduated from Tottenville High School in Staten Island, New York, and then earned her Associate's Degree in Applied Science in 2005, and a Bachelor's of Health Administration in 2009 from New York City College of Technology. Currently, she is attending courses towards an MS in Health Management from the College of Staten Island, part of CUNY. Cat utilizes her clinical dental hygiene license in a private practice on Staten Island, New York. She is also an adjunct lecturer at New York City College of Technology (NYCCT), CUNY, where she instructs students who are attending courses in the dental hygiene program. Cat also holds certifications in local anesthesia and nitrous oxide administration. She also holds an advisory role with Colgate-Palmolive. She enjoys offering her time in a voluntary capacity, having recently volunteered on Veterans Day at NYCCT, which offers free dental services to veterans; and "Dentistry from the heart", which offers free dental services to underprivileged individuals. In the past she has often assisted at the Jacob Javits Convention Center during the Greater New

York Dental Convention. She received the William Golterman Service Award for her volunteer work in 1998. This is an annual award presented to junior high school students who distinguish themselves by helping others. Cat has always shown a great interest in the dental field. She began working from a very early age as a dental assistant. Her childhood dentist had a profound influence in her life and career. She continues to work with this first, influential dentist. She enjoys working in this field in every capacity possible and will continue to strive to broaden her knowledge and expertise in her chosen career. She lives on the South Shore of Staten Island, New York, with her husband and two sons. Cat enjoys nothing more than spending time with her family. After dinner walks have become a tradition with her boys, who love the outdoors.

Lenny Nathan, BBA

Lenny received his BBA in Marketing/Advertising from Baruch College in New York City. His plan was to enter a business career in advertising. His career path changed, and he worked in television for a number of years before becoming a Unit Manager in 1979, at ABC Sports. He eventually excelled to the level of Senior Production Executive at ABC Sports where he worked on several television productions including the Olympics, Triple Crown Horse Racing, Monday Night Football, the Super Bowl, ABC's Wide World of Sports, among others. In 2003, he left television to become more involved in his adopted community of Rockland County, and perfect his golf game. He became involved in the local ambulance corps and became an EMT. He then became an Ambulance Corps instructor. He was dissatisfied with how EMTs received training. He started his own company, HealthSav LLC, which is an American Heart Association (AHA) Training Center. He currently runs HealthSav LLC and has been Regional EMT Faculty for the AHA for around 10 years. His most impressive accomplishments were working as a volunteer EMT for nine years. His certifications include: EMT, Basic Life Support, CPR Instructor and Training Center Coordinator. He has received AHA regional faculty national awards. Prior to becoming an EMT, he had a 30-year career at ABC Sports as a Production Executive where he held several Emmy nominations. His volunteer work includes serving on the Board of Directors for the Meals on Wheels program in Rockland County, New York. For more information visit: https://www.healthsav.com/.

Lucia Perez-Kleine, MA, LCAT, ATR-BC, LMHC

Lucia is a graduate of University of Florida and Florida Southern College, where she double majored in Studio Art and Psychology. She later moved to New York City to obtain her MA in Art Therapy at New York University (2006). Since then, she has been working with patients in psychiatric units who suffer from severe mental illnesses. She leads art therapy, verbal psychotherapy and psychoeducation-based groups. In 2014, she completed another master's program in Mental Health Counseling, also from New York University. Additional postgraduate studies include in-depth trauma studies at Columbia University's affiliated International Trauma Studies Program, as well as advanced training in verbal psychotherapy at New York Counseling and Clinical Social Work Institute. Currently, Lucia continues hospital work on an inpatient psychiatric unit and sees clients in her private psychotherapy practice in New York City. She is grateful for her loving and supportive family and to be doing work that she finds intellectually stimulating, impassioning and deeply gratifying.

Robert Peterman, DMD, MDS

Robert completed his dental degree at the University of Pennsylvania and completed a dental specialty residency in Orthodontics at Rutgers University. After graduation in 2014, he completed the board certification process to become a Diplomate of the American Board of Orthodontics. Only one in three orthodontists are board certified. He is currently the owner of a private orthodontic practice, Somerset Orthodontic Specialists, with two locations-one in Somerville, New Jersey, and one in Hillsborough, New Jersey. Robert has earned a reputation in New Jersey as one of the top orthodontists, winning multiple awards including being named New Jersey's Favorite Kids Doc. Robert regularly volunteers in his local community where he runs food drives for animal shelters, donates to charitable foundations and provides dental health education to elementary schools. Robert is a native of Staten Island, New York. He currently lives in New Jersey with his wife Natasha and two children, Robbie and Charlotte. For more information visit: https://www.somersetorthospecialists.com/.

Marita Powell, DO

Marita is the Osteopathic Director of Medical Education and the Director of Osteopathic Recognition for the Internal Medicine and Family Medicine Residencies and the Medical Student Program at United Health Services Hospitals, Inc. in Johnson City, New York. She is an Assistant Clinical Professor for State University of New York (SUNY) Upstate Medical University. Dr. Powell received her Doctor of Osteopathic Medicine from the New York College of Osteopathic Medicine and completed her osteopathic internship at Massapequa General Hospital, Long Island, New York, and her residency in Family Medicine at United Health Services Hospitals, Inc. She is board-certified in Family Medicine and Osteopathic Manipulative Medicine and was also a Licensed Registered Pharmacist. She has been a member of many organizations including the AOA, AMA, ACOFP, AAFP and the New York State Broome County Medical Society. Dr. Powell has given numerous lectures on both the local and national level pertaining to Family Medicine, Communications, Ethics and Osteopathic Manipulative Medicine. She is the author of a book entitled, "Just a Glance through the Window" written about her internship and published for teaching communications and bioethics to healthcare professionals in training. She is also a published poet. She enjoys spending time with family, cooking, swimming and acrylic painting. Dr. Powell resides in Conklin, New York, with her husband, also an osteopathic family physician, and their two sons.

Lauren B. Schwartz, MA, CCC-SLP

Lauren is a nationally certified and New York State licensed Speech-Language Pathologist and holds a Certificate of Clinical Competence from the American Speech Language Hearing Association. She earned her BS from Ithaca College as a Teacher of Speech and Hearing Handicapped and an MS from St. John's University in Speech-Language Pathology. Lauren has been employed as a Speech-Language Pathologist for 15 years with the NYC Department of Education with a focus on the elementary population with speech-language impairments, learning disabilities and autism. She is trained in PROMPT (PROMPTS for restructuring Oral Muscular Phonetic Targets) and the Orton-Gillingham Approach to reading instruction. Her clinical experiences include providing services in the home, clinic, preschool and rehabilitation setting and working with infants through early adulthood.

Rachel Schwartz, MA, MT-BC, LCAT, CASAC

Rachel is a Board Certified Music Therapist, Licensed Creative Arts Therapist, Credentialed Alcohol and Substance Abuse Counselor and Austin Vocal Psychotherapist. Ms. Schwartz graduated with a BA in Music and a minor in Psychology from Tulane University, New Orleans, Louisiana. She obtained her master's in music therapy at New York University. She has worked as a group psychotherapist at Mount Sinai Hospital in New York City on the inpatient psychiatric units for nine years and overall has worked on inpatient psychiatry for more than 10 years. She works predominantly with adults but has extensive experience working with the Mental Illness Chemical Addiction/Abuse (MICA), geriatric, children and adolescent populations in the inpatient psychiatric setting. Rachel also sees clients individually in her private practice. She is a member of the American Music Therapy Association (AMTA). She also has post-graduate training in the Diane Austin Vocal Psychotherapy Method. She has presented at the Mid-Atlantic Region of the AMTA Conference on Mindfulness as well as at Beth Israel Hospital's Louis Armstrong Center for Music and Medicine Symposium on substance use, misuse and dependence.

Maria Serrano-Miranda, MS, OTR/L

Maria is a certified occupational therapist assistant (COTA) and graduated with an associate's degree from Union County College in Scotch Plains, New Jersey. She continued her studies in occupational therapy and obtained her combined BS/MS degree to become a certified and licensed occupational therapist (OTR/L) at Dominican College of Blauvelt, New York. Maria has over 25 years of experience in the Occupational Therapy field, working with both adults and children. She is a senior occupational therapist in the NYC Department of Education and currently practices in a Staten Island elementary school. Maria volunteers in many local and community board activities. She truly believes that when you help someone in any way it will make a positive difference.

Robin Solomon, DVM

Robin is a graduate of Cornell University College of Veterinary Medicine. She is an associate veterinarian at a small animal hospital outside of Albany, New York. In her practice, she diagnoses and treats medical problems and provides preventative care to dogs and cats. The accomplishment that she is most proud of is her ability to connect with a wide variety of clients and provide the best care possible for each pet. She volunteers with a number of local cat and dog rescue organizations that are dedicated to limiting pet overpopulation and placing animals in forever homes.

James Spencer Verner, MS, RN

Spencer is a South Carolinian by birth. He was born in Spartanburg and raised in Newberry. After graduating high school, he joined the US Navy. He served as a hospital corpsman for four years. He was trained as a basic laboratory technician and a member of the Mobile Medical Readiness Team in Japan where he was introduced to Buddhism. When he completed his term in the Navy, Spencer continued his studies at the College of Charleston, where he double majored in psychology and philosophy. After graduating with his BS in Psychology, he moved to New York where he worked as a phlebotomist at various hospitals and clinics on Long Island. Seven years later, he returned to Charleston where he continued his studies in clinical counseling and nursing attaining a BSN from the Medical College of South Carolina. He continued his studies in psychiatric nursing and completed an MSN degree in 2010. He is continuing his studies in ethic-focused nursing practice, where he continues to pursue work in providing care to minorities and underserved patients and their families. He has worked in various psychiatric and detoxification centers, as well as, units specializing in stroke, neurological injury and epilepsy. Spencer also enjoys reading, writing, photography and travel. He is currently enjoying a fulfilling career as a private nurse.

CHAPTER 1

Surgical Technologist

Mark Fusco, CST

Education:	High School diploma	
	Surgical tech training program	<1-2 years
License:	Certified Surgical Technologist (CST) credential or the Tech in Surgery - Certified (TS-C) credential	
Median Income:	$47,300 (range, $32,870 - $69,170)*	

Differential shift (evenings, overnights), overtime and location will dictate salary.

Why I Became a Surgical Technologist

There is an old saying "life is a journey, not a destination." This is a difficult concept, especially when you are younger. You tend to view life in terms of age-oriented goals... when I am 25, I should have this... when I turn 40, I should have accomplished that. When these goals are not met – anger, frustration and sometimes depression occur. When you are older you realize age is just a number and life is a continual process of growth. When I was younger, I had no idea where I wanted my life to go. I bounced around from (what I felt at the time) were meaningless jobs. In my life I have been a clothing associate in a major department store, a mail clerk for a large Wall Street law firm, a timekeeper for an international shipping firm, a nurse's aide, a banquet cook and a pastry chef. For a brief time, I even worked in a Veterinarian's office handling exotic animals.

Now I am a surgical technologist. What a long and interesting trip it has been! Looking back at all the people I have met and the experiences I have had that helped shape me, I thank them all and I am extremely grateful to have known them.

This is a very important book. It fills a much-needed gap, exposing you to many opportunities in the medical field. You can also think of it as a life manual. Choosing a career can seem daunting, but remember, "You can change careers. Never feel like you are stuck." If a job doesn't feel right, move on and try something else, until it *does* feel right. When you are 50 years old with a family to support, it is much harder to switch gears. Now is the time to experiment. When you buy a t-shirt and a pair of jeans, you do not expect to wear them for the rest of your life. So why do people feel the need to stay in the same job their entire lives? I wish all of you well on your journey through life. Remember to laugh, love, and most of all explore as many different avenues as you can.

Overview

A drunk driver strikes a 19-year-old girl on her way home from college. An ambulance rushes her to the nearest emergency room. The doctors quickly realize she has massive internal injuries and is going into shock. They rush her into the operating room (OR). A flurry of activity begins. The anesthesiologist is desperately trying to put in intravenous (IV) lines, which serve to infuse medications, blood products and fluids. The trauma surgeon and his/her medical residents are deciding on their best course of action, nurses are getting medications and supplies and assisting in any way they can. Medical students are nervous and uncertain what to do... they just stand there. You, the surgical technologist, are alone in one part of the OR... your adrenaline is pumping, you are probably sweating, as you desperately struggle to set up your instruments to begin the surgery... you have about two minutes (it would normally take 20 minutes). The anesthesiologist yells out, "She's crashing," the surgeon asks if you are ready. You say yes—you have to be—any delay on your part would have a fatal result. The surgery lasts about three to four hours. Things went well. The bleeding has stopped, internal injuries are repaired, her vital signs (e.g., blood pressure, breathing rate, pulse) are stable. She will survive. You have helped give this girl back to her family. The doctor turns to you, smiles, and says, "good job." A sense of pride and accomplishment which you have never felt before swells within you. Welcome to the exciting world of Surgical Technology.

The Bureau of Labor Statistics predicts a 9% employment growth with 9,700 new jobs for Surgical Technologists between 2018-2028. Those individuals completing an accredited program will have the best job opportunities. The opportunities for the surgical technologist are as diverse as they are exciting. Do you want the rush of working at a major trauma hospital where victims of motor vehicle accidents or ruptured aneurysms come crashing through the door, or do you prefer a slower pace, working in a plastic surgeon's surgical suite, where you will be involved in every step, from cleaning and sterilizing your own instruments to being the surgeons first assistant? Do you dream of living in exciting cities and exotic locales, or like to travel and experience practice in different areas of the country? Then you can become a traveling tech. As a traveling tech, you would fill in for techs on a leave of absence from their job. Perhaps you are a humanitarian at heart, then you could work with Doctors without Borders, traveling to impoverished countries performing surgeries ranging from cleft palates to broken bones. The possibilities are endless, but you may think, "Can I make a living doing this?" Yes, you certainly can. The national pay average for a surgical tech is $23.58 per hour (about $49,040 annually). Eighty percent of surgical techs earn between $32,000 and $64,800. However, this is just a guide. In extremely rural areas salaries tend to be toward the lower end of the pay scale, but in major cities and metropolitan areas they are significantly higher. It is not unusual for an OR tech (also called a scrub tech) in a large city with 10 years of experience to make almost double the national average. Salaries are contingent upon many factors such as the size of the hospital, demand for scrub techs, and/or whether the hospital is unionized or not. Also, in most hospitals there is the opportunity for overtime, and "taking call." When you "take call," you are at home, but available to come in at a moment's notice for a possible emergency surgery. These are instances where you can greatly increase your base salary. I mentioned the idea of becoming a traveling tech. Hospitals that hire travelers usually need them desperately to fill in for their missing employees (e.g., someone out sick for surgery, maternity leave), and they pay well above base salary as well as a stipend for living expenses. If you are interested in the security of a government job, the United States (U.S.) Public Health Service or Veterans Administration (VA) hires surgical techs. As a government employee, salaries are on a government pay scale with yearly increases, and you receive a decent pension when you retire.

Nationwide, surgeries are on the rise, especially with the aging population requiring health and surgical care. Your career will never become obsolete and cannot be outsourced.

Specialties and Subspecialties

The type of surgery dictates the specialties where a scrub tech would work, including: orthopedics, obstetrics and gynecology, cardiothoracic, trauma, adult versus pediatric, general, neurosurgery, oral and facial, plastic surgery, otolaryngology (ear, nose and throat), urology, vascular surgery, to name some of the more common types of surgeries. Other "specialties" include the setting of the procedure, which would be either ambulatory (without staying overnight in a hospital) or in-patient. Then, as mentioned, there are traveling techs, versus techs that work in one hospital, or group of hospitals within a health-system.

Requirements

Training programs range from less than a year to two years. If you attend a two-year program you could obtain an associate's degree (at community colleges and vocational schools) or attend a nondegree program at a university. If you do not attend a two-year program you might graduate with a certificate. Some hospitals sponsor Surgical Tech programs to train employees who are working in less-skilled and lower-paying jobs. This is how I started as an OR Tech. Surgical tech program tuition costs vary. The Surgical Tech profession is formally regulated in a few states. Currently these states include Idaho, Indiana, Massachusetts, New Jersey, New York, South Carolina, Tennessee and Texas. To practice in these states, surgical techs must obtain nationally recognized certification and complete continuing education (CE) throughout their career. Many healthcare professions require certification and completion of continuing education throughout their career.

The surgical tech curriculum for certification includes both classroom (known as "didactic") training and clinical (or experiential) training. Classroom subjects include anatomy, biology, learning medical terminology (medical words), physiology (how the body works) and pharmacology (how drugs work). In the U.S., recognized certifications are the Certified Surgical Technologist (CST) credential from The National Board of Surgical Technology and Surgical Assisting, and the Tech in Surgery – Certified (TS-C) credential from the National Center for Competency Testing.

The medical field as a whole offers excellent career opportunities, and surgical technology affords you to be on the front lines of it all. Some have compared surgeons to fighter pilots in the military. If this is the case, then the surgical technologist is the flight engineer, ensuring everything runs smoothly from take-off to landing. If you are looking for a career which is mentally challenging, emotionally rewarding and has more thrills than a roller-coaster ride, then think about surgical technology. It just might be right for you.

A Day in the Life of a Surgical Technologist

The Surgical Technologist is an integral part of the OR team which consists of the surgeon (and possibly medical residents), an anesthesiologist and a circulating nurse. The circulating nurse provides the interface between sterile and non-sterile areas within the OR. Circulating nurses work in every OR, in every hospital across the country. They assist in every surgical discipline including, but not limited to Orthopedics, Cardiothoracic, Neurosurgery, Vascular, Plastic Surgery, Obstetrics and Gynecology and General Surgery. The role of the scrub tech is varied and the scrub tech has many responsibilities. However, we can summarize the scrub tech's main responsibilities into two very important functions: 1) setting up the OR prior to surgical procedures and 2) handling the instrumentation that the operating team uses during the surgery. The scrub tech must maintain the sterile field during the surgery (which minimizes post-operative infections). Every day is exciting and different. One day you may be working on a total knee replacement operation, which moves at an intense pace where instruments may number in the hundreds or thousands (and yes, you will learn them all). The next day you may be assisting in an aneurysm clipping in the brain, where everything moves very slowly. Any misstep on the surgeons' part, or yours, could have a fatal result. These are the physical mechanics of the job. However, your most important function in the OR is to maintain a calm and confident environment at all times. The surgeons have an awesome responsibility. They have someone's life in their hands. The surgeons have a big responsibility and they have no one to turn to. It is all up to them. I can tell you from personal experience, having a trauma come crashing through the door, the surgeons may not show it, but they are nervous. If they see you and have confidence in you, they will relax and breathe easier. Having this confidence increases the possibility for a successful surgical result.

Career Outlook

The U.S. News and World Report ranks Surgical Technologists as #18 in the Best Health Care Support Jobs, and #100 in 100 Best Jobs. Surgical Technologists have a relatively low 2.2% unemployment rate.

Search and Explore

Commission on Accreditation of Allied Health Education Programs
https://www.caahep.org/Students/Program-Info/Surgical-Technology.aspx

The National Board of Surgical Technology and Surgical Assisting
http://nbstsa.org/

Association of Surgical Technologists
http://www.ast.org

Cross Country TravCorps
https://www.crosscountrytravcorps.com/jobs/p-surgical-tech-operating-room-tech

American Traveler
https://www.americantraveler.com/nursing-specialties/operating-room

Similar Careers

Emergency Medical Technician

Certified Registered Nurse Anesthetist

Operating Room Nurse

Medical Assistant

Patient Care Assistant

Surgeon

CHAPTER 2

Pharmacist

Mary Choy, PharmD, BCGP, FASHP

Education:	Bachelor's Degree	4 years
	Doctor of Pharmacy Degree (PharmD)	4 years
	OR	
	Undergraduate	2 years
	Doctor of Pharmacy Degree (PharmD)	4 years
License:	Registered Pharmacist (RPh)	
Optional:	Residency/Fellowship	1 - 2 years
	Board Certification	
Median Income:	$126,120 (range, $87,420 - $159,410)	

Why I Became a Pharmacist

I knew I wanted to be a pharmacist since I was in my teens, a life-changing idea from my mom became my dream career. I was accepted into an accelerated pharmacy program and like most individuals, my first exposure to the profession was at a community pharmacy. During my first year in pharmacy school, I applied to multiple pharmacies for a job, but they wanted someone who was in their third year. Thus, I landed my first pharmacy job the old-fashioned way...I walked from pharmacy to pharmacy with my resume and after many rejections, finally an independent pharmacy hired me. I saw how the community pharmacist worked and the impact he made with the public, which solidified my interest in the profession. I was fascinated with the way medications worked and queried our pharmacist whenever I had the chance. A pharmacist works every day to make sure that patients' medications are accurate, safe and effective. The community pharmacist also conducts wellness clinics to ensure that patients are educated about optimal disease management such as asthma, high blood pressure, diabetes, and provides disease screening services. As I gained experience in community pharmacy, I was interested in challenging myself in other areas of healthcare. To enrich my experience, I was accepted into a competitive internship in the hospital where I assisted in preparing medications for inpatient orders and outpatient prescriptions. The hospital internship allowed me to have "hands-on" experience in preparing IV medications. During college, I knew that I didn't want to limit myself to one "type" of pharmacy practice. I wanted to have exposure to different pharmacy careers. By the time I graduated from pharmacy school, I was fortunate enough to have internship experiences from four different places: two independent pharmacies, one chain pharmacy, and one large medical center. Additionally, I had unique pharmacy school rotation experiences that focused on academia/teaching, compounding pharmacy and medical writing. I found it most rewarding to interact with patients and see their health improving. At this point, I knew that I wanted to continue my clinical training with a pharmacy residency. Pharmacy residencies typically last one to two years and the American Society of Health-System Pharmacists (ASHP) generally accredits them. After graduating from pharmacy school, I was elated to "match" with my first choice for the residency program and had the opportunity to take care of veterans who served our country. "Matching" in a pharmacy residency is similar to a medical residency that physicians undergo. Candidates and healthcare systems rank each other, and placements are made through a formal process. In my residency, I also had an adjunct faculty appointment at a college of pharmacy where I had the opportunity to teach two pharmacy courses. After my residency, I continued into an academic position as an Assistant Professor of Clinical Pharmacy where I found my passion in research, teaching and mentoring students. An additional passion was providing service to the underserved communities. My academic positions were dual appointments, which meant that I taught at the pharmacy school, and also served as a clinical pharmacist in a medical center. I started clinical programs (medication reconciliation, transitions of care; see glossary) at the medical centers to improve patient care. Because of all these experiences, I am who I am today: a pharmacist, an educator and a writer.

Overview

Pharmacists provide information about medications to patients and other healthcare professionals. As "medication experts," pharmacists are concerned with safeguarding the public's health in matters relating to medication use and distribution, and disease state management. Pharmacists also lead immunization clinics, manage diabetics blood sugar, provide medication therapy management (MTM; see glossary) and help smokers quit. Not only medication experts, pharmacists provide these and other services in addition to dispensing prescriptions. However, not all pharmacists dispense prescriptions. One must have a pharmacy license to dispense medications, but pharmacists do many other things including improving health outcomes, help hospitals decide which drugs will be available for inpatient use, and lower medication costs for patients.

If you think you are interested in a career in pharmacy, you can begin to prepare as early as middle school or high school. I personally know someone who was interested in becoming a pharmacist since elementary school. In addition to taking the math and science courses that are available to you, it would be a valuable experience to shadow a pharmacist. Shadowing allows you to see what a pharmacist does on a daily basis at his or her work setting. I would suggest shadowing a pharmacist in different disciplines, to see what interests you. In addition to shadowing a pharmacist, it is also a good idea to focus on taking math and science courses such as chemistry, biology and physics. Taking first aid classes may also help.

Specialties and Subspecialties

Pharmacy is a unique profession that is practiced in a wide range of settings: community/retail pharmacies, hospitals, large integrated health-systems, long-term care facilities, managed care, the pharmaceutical industry, nuclear, health informatics and government (Department of Defense, Department of Veterans Affairs, Indian Health Service, Public Health Service), to name a few.

The American College of Clinical Pharmacy (ACCP) defines clinical pharmacy as "a health science discipline in which pharmacists provide patient care that optimizes medication therapy and promotes health, wellness and disease prevention. Clinical pharmacists care for patients in all healthcare settings."

Pharmacists are the "medication experts" and the pharmacy profession's mission is to meet the pharmaceutical needs of the public. Pharmaceutical care is patient-centered and outcome-oriented that requires the pharmacist to work with the patient and the patients' healthcare providers to promote health, to prevent disease, and to assess, monitor, initiate and modify medication use so that pharmacotherapy is safe and effective.

Community/Retail Pharmacy: This is probably what most people associate with the pharmacy profession - community/retail pharmacists who dispense medications at independent pharmacies, chain stores or grocery stores. Pharmacists in these settings also oversee pharmacy students and pharmacy technicians.

Hospital Pharmacy: Hospital pharmacists face a varied number of responsibilities that include reviewing and approving appropriate medication orders that prescribers in the institution/hospital submit, dispensing medications, preparing IV medications, making non-sterile medications like certain liquid preparations for patient use in the hospital, overseeing pharmacy students and pharmacy technicians, making purchasing decisions, monitoring drug therapy and overseeing drug administration.

Clinical Pharmacy: Clinical pharmacists work directly with the physicians, nurses and other healthcare providers to provide optimal care. Some of the responsibilities include attending rounds on the medical team, assessing the status of the patient's health problems and determining whether the prescribed medications are optimally meeting the patient's needs, recognizing untreated health problems that could be improved or resolved with appropriate therapy, recommending changes to medication therapy, counseling the patient on how to best take his or her medications and serving as an educational resource for the medical team. Clinical pharmacists also provide clinical pharmacy services for the patients, such as medication reconciliation, transitions of care and antimicrobial stewardship. Clinical pharmacists may also be involved with helping decide which drugs are available on the hospital formulary (see glossary), by helping evaluate the medical literature (e.g., journal articles) and approved product label information, as well as monitoring and reporting on adverse drug reactions, as a member of the P & T Committee (see glossary).

Long-Term Care: Long-term care pharmacists generally have two career paths: one focuses on dispensing/management operations and the other on consultant services. The various long-term care settings include hospitals that own skilled nursing facilities, long-term care pharmacies, nursing homes and rehabilitation services. Consultant services include formalized, clinical, state mandated medication reviews to monitor for appropriate medication use.

Managed Care: Managed care pharmacists work for health plans and pharmacy benefit management (PBM, see glossary) companies. They perform a variety of functions that include drug formulary management, drug distribution and dispensing, patient safety monitoring, clinical program development, disease management programs and cost management. MTM (see glossary) may also be part of the responsibilities of a managed care pharmacist.

Pharmaceutical Industry: Industry pharmacists work in areas that include clinical research, drug safety, medical affairs, regulatory affairs, marketing, sales, medical/drug information, medical writing and education and training.

Nuclear Pharmacy: Nuclear pharmacists prepare and dispense radiopharmaceuticals which the medical profession uses in digital imaging scans such as magnetic resonance imaging (MRI), computerized tomography scans (CT) and other procedures in medical offices and hospitals. Nuclear pharmacists typically start their work day very early since the radiopharmaceuticals are administered to patients on the same day the pharmacist prepares them.

Health Informatics: Informatics pharmacists use technology to streamline patient care, medication safety, and focus on medication-related data. Projects include maintaining pharmacy computer systems and electronic health records, creating medication alerts, IV medication pump safety, barcode medication administration, to name a few.

Contract, Temporary or Hourly Pharmacy Careers: For pharmacists who are unable to commit to a specific area or have a limited amount of time to work, they can work on a contract basis until they find the best fit, or they can work part-time. Contract pharmacy careers offer flexibility in the schedule and allow pharmacists to experience different employers and work settings prior to making a long-term commitment. For pharmacists who like to travel around the country, there are also travel pharmacy positions.

Requirements

There are currently 143 colleges and schools of pharmacy in the U.S. that offer the Doctor of Pharmacy (Pharm.D.) as a first professional degree. To be admitted into pharmacy school, you must fulfill certain prerequisite class requirements which are usually achieved by having at least two years of specific undergraduate college study followed by four academic years of professional pharmacy study. While a bachelor's degree is not required for most pharmacy schools, some schools do give preference to those who have one. The required undergraduate courses usually include calculus, and basic sciences such as biology, general chemistry, organic chemistry, physics and microbiology. Other factors that pharmacy schools take into account for admission include work/volunteer experience in a pharmacy, hospital or healthcare setting, and three letters of recommendation. The Pharmacy College Admission Test (PCAT) score is either required or strongly preferred for most schools. Many schools also have a full day on-site interview process for prospective candidates.

If you know early on that you want to pursue pharmacy, then it is possible to go from high school to pharmacy school. Some pharmacy schools accept students immediately after they graduate from high school. These students can complete their pre-pharmacy and professional study within six years after high school, so they are referred to as "0-6" programs. In addition, there are many other pharmacy colleges and schools that offer "early assurance" also known as "early admission" for selected high school students. The similarities of the "early assurance" to the "0-6" program are that students who successfully complete the first two years of pre-professional study are guaranteed admission into the four-year professional pharmacy program. The "early assurance" programs are different from the "0-6" programs in that most students enrolled are admitted as "transfer" students after completing at least two years of college.

As part of the pharmacy curriculum, students also complete supervised work experiences, known as internships, in different settings such as hospitals, clinics, managed care companies and retail/outpatient pharmacies.

In order to dispense medications, a pharmacist must pass the North American Pharmacist Licensure Examination (NAPLEX) and Multistate Pharmacy Jurisprudence Examination (MPJE, also known as the state pharmacy law exam) and fulfill the licensing requirements for the state in which they want to work. This license is mandatory for those to dispense medications in either an outpatient (community) or inpatient (mostly hospitals) setting. New York State is the only state that also requires pharmacists to pass a compounding examination to become licensed. Each state may also have specific licensing requirements. Contact the specific state board of pharmacy for licensure requirements in each state. Visit: https://nabp.pharmacy/programs/ for more information.

All states require formal CE for pharmacists to renew their licenses. According to the Accreditation Council for Pharmacy Education (ACPE), continuing education "is a structured educational activity designed or intended to support the continuing development of pharmacists to maintain and enhance their competence." The variety of formats include – in-person, written, live webinar, self-paced learning or podcasts, which experts in the field deliver to pharmacists for their professional development.

Pharmacists may also choose to pursue board certifications through the Board of Pharmacy Specialties. There are currently 13 specialized care areas. These include: ambulatory care, cardiology, compounded sterile preparations, critical care, geriatrics, infectious diseases, nuclear, nutrition support, oncology, pediatric, pharmacotherapy, psychiatry and solid organ transplantation. Board certifications are not mandatory but may play a role in obtaining a clinical pharmacy position. Some positions will list board certifications as a job requirement. You can obtain more information on board certification at the Board of Pharmacy Specialties (https://www.bpsweb.org/).

Instead of, or in addition to a Pharmacy Residency, pharmacy students may also apply for a post-graduate one- or two-year Fellowship. These programs are mainly geared towards different aspects of pharmacy research, drug information, academia or medical affairs in the pharmaceutical industry. These programs often "pair-up" with a health-system (hospital/managed care plan) or a college of pharmacy to provide different opportunities for the applicant. Some Fellowships are also in managed care pharmacy.

A Day in the Life of a Pharmacist

I love being a pharmacist because of the impact that I make in my patients' lives. As a pharmacist working in academia and clinical pharmacy, every day is different and that's what makes it exciting. In addition to teaching at the college, professors have patient care responsibilities at their clinical site, engage in research and are involved in professional organizations. The three pillars of academia are: teaching, scholarship and service. An important balance of these three pillars is imperative for success in the academic world.

On certain days at the college campus, I am giving lectures to pharmacy students, attending faculty meetings, writing exam questions, preparing for lectures and meeting/mentoring students. Teaching has always been my passion and I have found it fulfilling to prepare the next generation of pharmacists and teach healthcare professionals and the public. On other days at the clinical practice site, my morning begins by reviewing the patients' medical charts, participating on medical rounds through the multidisciplinary healthcare team and making appropriate medication recommendations to the medical team (changes in medications, doses, frequency of dosing, discontinuation of medications). I also precept pharmacy students at the hospital and meet with them to ensure that they are prepared for the multidisciplinary rounds (a preceptor is an experiential educator; see glossary). Through multidisciplinary rounds, different disciplines such as medical, pharmacy, nursing and social work come together to coordinate patient care, establish daily goals and plan for potential patient transfer or discharge from the hospital. This is a patient-centered model of care that is instrumental in improving the quality, safety and patient experience. Many hospital statistics indicate that using multidisciplinary rounds reduces patients' lengths of hospital stay. Throughout the day, there will be scheduled meetings, and by late afternoon, students will typically present their assignments (disease state presentations, case presentations and drug information questions) to me. Additionally, one of the clinical pharmacy services that I helped establish was discharge medication counseling where my students and I are involved in improving patient safety and the hospitals' initiatives with transitions of care (see glossary). After the students and I review the patient's discharge medication regimen, the outpatient pharmacy fills the prescriptions. We then counsel the patient at the bedside. In addition to providing patients with verbal information, they also receive a medication sheet noting the times at which they should take each medication. They also receive an information sheet for each drug. Throughout the day, we communicate with physicians, nurses, pharmacists and students. The day is busy, and I love that I am able to teach and make a difference for patients.

The commitments, opportunities and learning continue after the workday. On certain evenings, I attend pharmacy organization board meetings, medical and pharmacy CE meetings. I am fortunate to have the opportunity to serve the profession in leadership roles on the state and national level. I encourage everyone involved in pharmacy to be fully engaged. It is important to advocate and make a difference. At CE meetings, I fulfill my obligations for the mandatory CE requirements for relicensure, learn about new medical advances, network with other practitioners and am inspired. As a pharmacist, it is important to continually reinvent yourself, stay competitive and network to achieve unique perspectives and inspiration. Pharmacy is not only a career to me, pharmacy is my life.

Career Outlook

According to the U.S. News and World Report, Pharmacists rank #55 in 100 Best Jobs, #22 in Best Healthcare Jobs, and #21 in Best Paying Jobs. The Bureau of Labor Statistics projects 0% (little or no change) employment growth for pharmacists between 2018 and 2028. Pharmacists have a 2.1% unemployment rate; the best-paid 25% of pharmacists made $142,710, while the lowest-paid 25% made $110,310. In May 2018, the median annual wage for pharmacists was $126,120.

Search and Explore

Accreditation Council for Pharmacy Education (ACPE)
   http://www.acpe-accredit.org

Academy of Managed Care Pharmacy (AMCP)
   http://www.amcp.org

American Association of Colleges of Pharmacy (AACP)
   http://www.aacp.org

American College of Clinical Pharmacy (ACCP)
   http://www.accp.com

American Pharmacists Association (APhA)
   http://www.apha.org

American Society of Health-System Pharmacists (ASHP)
   http://www.ashp.org

American Society of Consultant Pharmacists (ASCP)
   http://www.ascp.com

Board of Pharmacy Specialties (BPS)
   http://www.bpsweb.org

National Association of Boards of Pharmacy
   https://nabp.pharmacy/programs/

National Association of Chain Drug Stores (NACDS)
   http://www.nacds.org

Albert E. Fellowships 101: Q&A with a Residency and Fellowship Director
   https://www.pharmacytimes.com/publications/career/2015/pharmacycareers_
   february2015/fellowships-101

Definitions of Pharmacy Residencies and Fellowships. Published 1987.
   https://www.ashp.org/-/media/assets/policy-guidelines/docs/endorsed-documents/
   definitions-of-pharmacy-residencies-and-fellowships.ashx/

Similar Careers

Physician

Physician Assistant

Nurse Practitioner

Pharmacy Technician

CHAPTER 3

Pharmacy Technician

Zachary Green, CPhT

Education:	High School diploma / General Education Diploma (GED)	<1-2 years
	OR	
	Bachelor's Degree	4 years
Certification:	Certified Pharmacy Technician (CPhT) through the Pharmacy Technician Certification Board (PTCB)	
Median Income:	$34,020 (range, $22,740 - $48,010)	

Why I Became a Pharmacy Technician

I have always been interested in healthcare. During the first couple of years of college I did not know exactly what I wanted to do. I knew that promoting health and wellbeing would be a part of what made me happy. It was during this time that I discovered becoming a pharmacy technician had the least number of requirements to work compared to other health professions and I saw it as somewhat of a stepping stone into our vast healthcare system. After working as a pharmacy technician I found a passion in this as a career, not just a job, I found myself drawn to the entire profession of pharmacy to improve the wellbeing of the public, and have since made a career in the profession of pharmacy. Although I no longer work in a pharmacy as a technician, I am employed at the Pharmacy Technician Certification Board (PTCB). At PTCB, I work with passionate educators of pharmacy technicians as well as employers of pharmacy technicians committed to one standard of pharmacy technician certification, education and training for the front line – pharmacy technicians. I obtained a bachelor's degree in order to work in the public policy field, related to the pharmacy profession, but in order to be a pharmacy technician, you must have a high school diploma or GED.

Overview

Pharmacy technicians are an integral part of the entire healthcare team. Pharmacy Technicians assist the pharmacist in dispensing prescription medication directly to patients. Assisting the pharmacist happens across all practice settings from independently owned community pharmacies, large community chain pharmacies, grocery stores with pharmacies, mail order facilities and hospitals. A pharmacy technician may be employed in many areas. Technician responsibilities differ in each practice setting but below are examples:

- Inputting patient, insurance and prescription information

- Filling and labeling medication vials

- Sterile and non-sterile compounding of medications and solutions

- Specialty pharmacy medications (see glossary)

- Inventory management

- Answering phones (in some states pharmacy technicians are also able to take new or refill prescription information over the phone)

Specialties and Practice Settings

Some pharmacy technicians can have a concentrated focus and specialize within certain areas of pharmacy such as sterile compounding (making IV's), MTM, 340B, insurance, patient assistance programs, information technology, and inventory management or supply chain/logistics. 340B pertains to a U.S. Federal Drug Discount Program that requires drug manufacturers to provide outpatient drugs to eligible healthcare organizations and covered entities at significantly reduced prices. The program only covers certain drugs and hospitals. These can include cancer drugs, children's hospitals, and cancer hospitals. Since hospitals treat a mix of different types of insured patients, technicians who have this role help the hospitals with the acquisition, maintenance, use and billing of these drugs. Not only can technicians work in these areas but they can also manage a team of technicians and teach other technicians at educational institutions. In recent years, there has also been an increase in pharmacy technician involvement on state boards of pharmacy where they serve as a technician voice in a state regulatory environment. Although pharmacy technicians work in a variety of settings, performing similar duties across each, some technicians perform different tasks in different practice settings. Below are some of these examples.

Nursing home, long term care facilities, home infusion: Pharmacy technicians working in this area of pharmacy assist the pharmacist in dispensing medications to nursing units generally in a unit-dose (or single dose) form. Technicians also must stock automated dispensing cabinets (ADCs; see glossary) where other health professionals, such as nurses or physicians, can obtain medications for their patients. Pharmacy technicians working in this environment have limited patient interaction but are integral in medication preparation and delivery. There are aspects of this setting that may include patient interaction such as outpatient services (similar to the community setting) or obtaining patient medication histories.

Sterile and non-sterile compounding of medications and solutions: Pharmacy technicians also perform sterile and non-sterile compounding. Technicians can be responsible for admixing (making or preparing) IV medications for delivery as well as for non-sterile topical or oral use. Sterile compounding of IV medications often includes narcotics for pain management, antibiotics, pressors to main blood pressure in a normal range, anti-seizure drugs and cancer chemotherapy.

Chemotherapy: Chemotherapy for cancer treatment is a specialized area within the sterile compounding role of the pharmacy technician. This often requires additional training, and this may be a sole responsibility of technicians in certain practice settings.

Medication history or reconciliation: Pharmacy technicians can perform medication history or reconciliation and as of 2017 is a newer, expanded role for technicians. Technicians in this role interact with patients obtaining their medication history and inputting this information into a patient's chart for physicians, pharmacists and other healthcare team members to review.

In the Community setting: which also can be called retail or ambulatory, consists of working in small independent, large community chain or grocery stores that contain a pharmacy. Pharmacy technicians working in this environment interact with patients very frequently.

Medication Therapy Management (MTM): Technicians have played an increasing role in this aspect of pharmacy where the pharmacist consults with patients taking multiple medications. The technician can be responsible for reviewing a patient profile to alert the pharmacist for the need of a consultation and schedule patient appointments with the pharmacist for the consultation.

Immunizations: Licensed pharmacists or pharmacy interns traditionally have administered immunizations. Recently, the Idaho, Rhode Island, and Utah Boards of Pharmacy have allowed pharmacy technicians, after proper accredited training, and appropriate supervision, to administer vaccines. Other states are trying to pass immunization administration legislation for pharmacy technicians.

In December 2017, PTCB launched their advanced certificate program, the Certified Compounded Sterile Preparation Technician (CSPT®) for any certified technicians wanting to obtain a more advanced level of training in a particular area. Six additional certificate programs are in the development process in the following areas: Technician Product Verification (Tech-Check-Tech), Medication History, Controlled Substance Diversion Prevention, Billing and Reimbursement, Hazardous Drug Management and Immunizations.

Requirements

Currently there is no national standard to work as a pharmacy technician nor is there a national standard for educating pharmacy technicians. However, there are various avenues to become a pharmacy technician. Some states require registration or licensure with the board of pharmacy, formal education, CE and/or national certification distinguished by the credential CPhT. Employers will require, at minimum, what the state requires, but may have additional requirements such as previous work experience in the field or a specific national certification. To become a pharmacy technician, one should look to their state board of pharmacy for the requirements and then look to what a future employer might require. I would recommend obtaining a formal pharmacy technician training program that is accredited by the ASHP and Accreditation Council for Pharmacy Education (ACPE) and then obtaining a national certification that all practice settings and all fifty states recognize. A PTCB certified pharmacy technician is required to earn 20 hours of pharmacy technician specific CE every two years in order to maintain the certification. Of the 20 hours, one hour is required to cover pharmacy law as well as one required hour of patient safety.

A Day in the Life of a Pharmacy Technician

Because of my current role as associate director of partnership development at PTCB, my day in the life as a pharmacy technician is quite different than that of a traditional setting. I serve as the primary liaison to pharmacy technician educators and employers participating in the PTCB Advocate Programs. These programs provide several benefits to employers and educators of pharmacy technicians who either require or encourage PTCB Certification. In this role, I work to orient new participants of the Advocate Programs as well as build new relationships. My day-to-day tasks include answering emails regarding questions related to the PTCB Certification Program, as it pertains to educators such as providing school performance reporting and to employers in ways such as assisting with mass verification of certification to determine if pharmacy technicians are in compliance. I also attend state and national pharmacy association conferences across the U.S. I exhibit on trade show floors representing PTCB to promote the PTCB Certification Program and to build the advocate programs by networking with employers and educators.

In my previous role as a pharmacy technician in a hospital, I performed many of the various tasks around assisting the pharmacist in filling prescriptions. These tasks involved restocking ADCs throughout the hospital in various nursing units and on all hospital floors. I also performed cart-fill where technicians pulled daily medication for patients in the hospital for a pharmacist to check. After the pharmacists check the cart-fill, pharmacy technicians delivered the medications to the patient's rooms. To me, the most enjoyable task however, was working in the IV room where I compounded sterile products to be delivered in cart-fill, and as needed. This also involved compounding IV medications for surgeries, controlled substance IV narcotic medications, as well as various maintenance IV medications. The shifts I worked were generally eight hours in the afternoon. The work varied daily but I could always complete my tasks in those eight hours. If I could not complete my work during my shift due to a heavier workload (e.g., more patients needing these medications), I could pass it to the person covering my assigned area of the pharmacy on the next shift.

Career Outlook

U.S. News and World Report Best Jobs ranks Pharmacy Technician as #92 in Best Jobs, and #16 in Best Health Care Support Jobs, noting a median salary of $31,750 with most individuals working in pharmacies/drug stores and hospitals. The Bureau of Labor Statistics projects 7% employment growth for pharmacy technicians between 2018 and 2028, a 2.1% unemployment rate, and approximately 31,500 new jobs in this ten-year timeframe.

Search and Explore

American Society of Health-System Pharmacists (ASHP) - technicians
https://www.ashp.org/Pharmacy-Technician/About-PharmacyTechnicians/Pharmacy-

Technician-Career-Overview American Pharmaceutical Association
http://www.pharmacist.com

American Association of Pharmacy Technicians (AAPT)
https://www.pharmacytechnician.com/

National Pharmacy Technician Association (NPTA)
http://www.pharmacytechnician.org/

National Associations of Boards of Pharmacy (NABP)
http://nabp.pharmacy

Pharmacy Technician certification Board (PTCB)
http://www.ptcb.org

Similar Careers

Dental Assistant

Medical Assistant

Medical Records and Health Information Technician

Medical Transcriptionist

Pharmacist

CHAPTER 4

Osteopathic Physician

Marita R. Powell, DO

Education:	Bachelor's Degree	4 years
	DO Degree	4 years
	Residency	3+ years (depending on specialty)
	Fellowship (optional)	3+ years (depending on specialty)
License:	National Board of Osteopathic Medical Examiners (NBOME)	
Median Income:	$208,000 (range, $200,000 - $500,000+)*	

income depends on specialty and geographic area; surgeons salary ranges from $255,000 to $500,000+)

Why I Became an Osteopathic Physician

During my undergraduate studies at the University of Rhode Island College of Pharmacy, I was most interested in learning about how drugs worked in the body and how drugs influenced treatment of diseases rather than the more technical aspects of compounding and filling actual prescriptions that physicians write. During the 1980s, Pharmacy School was a five-year program to obtain a bachelor's degree or one could study for two more years to obtain a Doctor of Pharmacy (PharmD) degree, where one could practice as a clinical pharmacist. I immediately gravitated toward becoming a clinical pharmacist but once I fully investigated it, I realized that even after seven years of study, and despite gaining much knowledge of medicine, I still could not diagnose or prescribe as a physician. However, while I was in school, I realized I would need to complete another two years for a PharmD, so this compelled me to do more research on how to become a medical doctor. I took a pharmacy law class that taught us about the different types of medical doctors who can write prescriptions. This is when I learned the term osteopathic physician or DO (will be explained later). Since I am from New England, the only physicians I had known were allopathic (MDs). My role model was my family physician who took care of my entire family, even my great grandmother. He was an MD by training and was very holistic in his approach to care. I knew I wanted my specialty to be family medicine, so I could take care of families through an emphasis of wellness and prevention. I knew drugs saved lives but could also have bad side effects and there was always a risk-benefit ratio to consider when taking medicines. I saw drugs save my grandfather's life many times since he suffered from heart failure, after having a heart attack in the 1970s. I also saw my aunt die from severe anemia from a drug that shut down her bone marrow after she took it for joint pain.

Once I understood what a DO was, I knew it was the kind of medical doctor I wanted to become. As a pharmacist, I felt like an expert in my drug knowledge to treat patients and knew that using this knowledge would help me be a better doctor, but I wanted to know what else I could do to help my patients. I knew that one's state of mind is connected to one's health and that some people can "worry" themselves into an ulcer or heart problems. I wanted to learn what "nondrug prescriptions" I could give my patients. I wanted to learn osteopathic manipulation.

Overview

Doctors of Osteopathic Medicine are physicians who practice in every medical specialty. Because of our unique philosophy, many of us choose the primary care fields of Family Medicine, Internal Medicine and/or Pediatrics. We have a holistic philosophy which means we are trained to treat the whole person, not just the body part. We consider the mind, body and spirit as components of both health and disease and realize the importance of prevention to maintain health.

Like our allopathic (MD) colleagues, we practice according to the best up-to-date science and use the newest innovative technologies available, and also consider options to complement pharmaceuticals and surgery.

There are more than 100,000 DOs in the U.S., practicing in every medical specialty. Currently one out of every four medical students are studying to become a DO. Osteopathic physicians have additional training in Osteopathic Manipulative Treatment (OMT) or Osteopathic Manipulative Medicine (OMM), in addition to the same training that allopathic physicians obtain. The profession often uses the terms interchangeably. By palpating the body's bones and soft tissues with our hands, we are able to diagnose, treat and prevent illness and injury.

Through OMT, DOs use their hands to diagnose illness and injury and encourage your body's natural tendency toward self-healing. When in school and training, DOs learn how the body's systems are interconnected and how each one affects the others.

During medical school, DOs receive special training in anatomy and palpation to learn techniques that affect a patient's musculoskeletal system, the body's interconnected system of nerves, muscles and bones. Using manipulation, DOs can effectively treat the muscles and joints to relieve pain, promote healing and increasing overall mobility.

DOs often use these manipulation skills for non-muscle skeletal disorders as well, like cardiac and pulmonary diseases. The osteopathic training emphasizes the importance of treating the cause of disease, not just the symptoms.

DOs can use OMT to complement, or even replace drugs or surgery. For example, if you are my patient and you see me for a tension headache, I can prescribe a pain medicine. Another option is that I can also palpate the muscles in your neck and check your leg length. I would then use OMT to eliminate your muscle spasm in your neck and back, correct your leg length so you stand straighter which could have been one of the causes of your tension headache. Then I would talk to you about prevention. These preventative tips could include good posture or not wearing a back pack over your shoulders so your headaches do not recur. I also do not want you to become dependent on pain medicines!

In the U.S., there are about three to four times as many allopathic (MD) medical schools as osteopathic (DO) medical schools. Many great physicians have graduated from U.S. osteopathic medical schools, U.S. allopathic medical schools and non-U.S. allopathic medical schools. When you research prospective medical schools, it would be helpful to look at school rankings, requirements for entrance such as grades, Medical College Admissions Test (MCAT) scores, success rates of passing medical board examinations, class size, student-teacher ratio, rotation placement and support.

Osteopathic Medical Education

Doctors of Osteopathy or Osteopathic Physicians in the U.S. receive medical training very similar to their allopathic colleagues (MDs), but DOs have additional training in OMT. After undergraduate education of usually four years, DOs and MDs attend four years of medical school followed by graduate medical education through internships and residencies. Residencies are generally three to four years and prepare the osteopathic physician to practice in any medical specialty, but many choose a primary care specialty because of the emphasis on holistic medicine. Both DOs and MDs pass comparable certification exams to obtain their medical licenses, and they can practice in fully accredited and licensed healthcare facilities.

Brief History of Osteopathic Medicine

Dr. Andrew Taylor Still is the Father of Osteopathy (1828-1917), the son of a Methodist minister and physician who studied medicine with his father. He lost family members to pneumonia and meningitis and became dissatisfied with the medicine of his time. He devoted his life to studying the human body and found alternative ways to treat disease. He founded the American School of Osteopathy (ASO) in Kirksville, Virginia in 1892. He said, "an osteopath is down-to-earth, observes the laws of nature and, acting as an engineer of human bodies, brings them back to life in order to restore their health." The philosophy of osteopathic medicine follows four principles: (1) the body as a unit; (2) structure and function are interrelated; (3) the body possesses self-regulatory mechanisms; and (4) the body has the inherent capacity to defend and repair itself.

Specialties and Subspecialties

Physician specialties are literally A to V, all requiring their own number of years of training but all starting with four years of medical school, followed by residency training years and possibly fellowship training years. There are over 120 medical specialties and subspecialties. Once a physician becomes "boarded" in their specialty, they have to maintain their expertise with continuing medical education (CME). This again depends on their chosen specialty.

For example, my specialty of Family Medicine requires three years of residency after medical school. With successful completion of residency, family doctors take a full day written exam. Once one successfully passes this, one receives initial board certification and then enters a maintenance of board certification process. The American Board of Family Medicine requires a family doctor to have 50 hours of CME per year, participate in simulated patient modules on family medicine topics and pass a full day exam every 10 years to maintain their Board certification. Likewise, for DOs, the American Osteopathic Board of Family Physicians requires similar CME, but their exam is every eight years and includes both a written and practical test in osteopathic manipulation. The bottom line... a medical career takes many years of training and a lifetime of study!

Specialties and subspecialties include:

- Abdominal Radiology
- Addiction Psychiatry
- Adolescent Medicine
- Adult Reconstructive Orthopedics
- Advanced Heart Failure and Transplant Cardiology
- Allergy and Immunology
- Anesthesiology
- Biochemical Genetics
- Blood Banking - Transfusion Medicine

- Cardiothoracic Radiology
- Cardiovascular Disease
- Chemical Pathology
- Child and Adolescent Psychiatry
- Child Abuse Pediatrics
- Child Neurology
- Clinical and Laboratory Immunology
- Clinical Cardiac Electrophysiology
- Clinical Neurophysiology

- Colon and Rectal Surgery
- Congenital Cardiac Surgery
- Craniofacial Surgery
- Critical Care Medicine
- Cytopathology
- Dermatology
- Dermatopathology
- Developmental (Behavioral Pediatrics)
- Emergency Medicine
- Endocrinology, Diabetes & Metabolism
- Endovascular Surgical Neuroradiology
- Family Medicine
- Family Practice
- Female Pelvic Medicine & Reconstructive Surgery
- Foot and Ankle Orthopedics
- Forensic Pathology
- Forensic Psychiatry
- Gastroenterology
- Geriatric Medicine (Family Medicine, Internal Medicine, Family Practice)
- Geriatric Psychiatry
- Hand Surgery (Orthopedics,

Plastic Surgery)
- Hematology (Internal Medicine, Pathology)
- Hematology and Oncology (Internal Medicine)
- Infectious Disease (Internal Medicine)
- Internal Medicine
- Internal Medicine (Pediatrics)
- Interventional Cardiology
- Medical Genetics
- Medical Microbiology (Pathology)
- Medical Toxicology (Emergency Medicine, Preventive Medicine)
- Molecular Genetic Pathology (Medical Genetics)
- Musculoskeletal Radiology (Diagnostic Radiology)
- Musculoskeletal Oncology
- Neonatal-Perinatal Medicine (Pediatrics)
- Nephrology (Internal Medicine)
- Neurological Surgery
- Neurology
- Neuromuscular Medicine (Neurology, Physical Medicine & Rehabilitation)

- Neuropathology
- Neuroradiology (Diagnostic)
- Nuclear Medicine
- Nuclear Radiology (Diagnostic)
- Obstetric Anesthesiology (Anesthesiology)
- Obstetrics and Gynecology
- Oncology (Internal Medicine)
- Ophthalmic Plastic and Reconstructive Surgery (Ophthalmology)
- Ophthalmology
- Orthopedic Sports Medicine Orthopaedic Surgery
- Orthopedic Surgery
- Orthopedic Surgery of the Spine Orthopaedic Surgery
- Orthopedic Trauma Orthopaedic Surgery
- Otolaryngology
- Otology - Neurotology (Otolaryngology)
- Pain Medicine (Anesthesiology, Neurology, Physical Medicine and Rehabilitation)
- Pathology (Anatomic and Clinical)
- Pediatric Anesthesiology (Anesthesiology)

- Pediatric Cardiology (Pediatrics)
- Pediatric Critical Care Medicine (Pediatrics)
- Pediatric Emergency Medicine (Emergency Medicine, Pediatrics)
- Pediatric Endocrinology (Pediatrics)
- Pediatric Gastroenterology (Pediatrics)
- Pediatric Hematology-Oncology (Pediatrics)
- Pediatric Infectious Diseases (Pediatrics)
- Pediatric Nephrology (Pediatrics)
- Pediatric Orthopedics Orthopedic Surgery
- Pediatric Otolaryngology
- Pediatric Pathology
- Pediatric Pulmonology (Pediatrics)
- Pediatric Radiology (Diagnostic)
- Pediatric Rheumatology (Pediatrics)
- Pediatric Sports Medicine (Pediatrics)
- Pediatric Surgery (General Surgery)
- Pediatric Transplant Hepatology (Pediatrics)
- Pediatric Urology (Urology)

- Pediatrics
- Physical Medicine and Rehabilitation
- Plastic Surgery
- Preventive Medicine
- Procedural Dermatology
- Psychiatry
- Pulmonary Disease (Internal Medicine)
- Pulmonary Disease and Critical Care Medicine (Internal Medicine)
- Radiation Oncology
- Radiology (Diagnostic)
- Rheumatology (Internal Medicine)
- Sleep Medicine

- Spinal Cord Injury Medicine (Physical Medicine & Rehabilitation)
- Sports Medicine Emergency Medicine, Family Medicine, Internal Medicine, Physical Medicine and Rehabilitation
- Surgical Critical Care
- General Surgery
- Thoracic Surgery
- Thoracic Surgery-Integrated
- Transplant Hepatology (Internal Medicine)
- Urology
- Vascular and Interventional Radiology (Diagnostic, General Surgery)

Requirements

To become a doctor, you need to study hard and obtain good grades. You should take challenging courses in high school including Science, Math and English. If you volunteer at a hospital, this can expose you to different medical fields and provide you with community service. Some hospitals will let you volunteer as early as 15 years of age, and as you advance towards college, you may be allowed to shadow doctors in different specialties like the Emergency Department (ED).

You can also look for summer programs like Medical Academy of Science and Health (MASH) Camp which is for eighth and ninth graders. MASH Camp lets you spend supervised time in a local hospital doing fun activities, learning about different health careers and educational requirements for those careers. When considering an application to medical school, a strong academic record is very important, but extracurricular activities show diversity and leadership skills, which are also important.

The application process to medical school is a multi-step process.

At the undergraduate level, many colleges/universities have different health profession organizations or pre-professional clubs that you should join. Most colleges/universities also have "pre-med" advisors that will counsel, guide and educate you through the application process. Many colleges/universities also have a pre-professional evaluation committee that checks your paperwork, interviews you and sends a committee letter on your behalf to the medical schools to which you apply. Before applying to colleges, check with your high school advisor who can help you. However most colleges list this information directly on their website under their pre-med or pre-health professional categories in the academic curriculum section.

Usually when you are between your third and fourth year in college, you can submit your medical school applications. The application process requires submitting a primary application, containing biographical information, grades and MCAT scores. The MCAT is a one-day exam testing your knowledge in many subjects such as chemistry, biology, physics, psychology, sociology, statistics and critical reading skills. That is why it is so important to study Science, Math and English. Medical schools not only want to see strong grades in these subjects, they want to see community service, exposure to medical fields, research, good communication skills and a diversity of interests. Once you submit your primary application, medical schools interested in you will require a secondary application. This application will have more questions to answer, but they are specific to that particular school. The medical school may then contact you for an interview.

My Personal Experience with Osteopathy

After completing Osteopathic medical school, I went on to become a Board Certified Family Physician. Taking care of family members of all ages including delivering babies, I was now able to apply my OMT skills to help many people address the causes of their disease and not just their symptoms. Then came my own disease - Rheumatoid Arthritis (RA). I was diagnosed in my late 40s and, of course, the arthritis affected my hands - the most precious tool an osteopath uses to perform OMT. Being a well-trained family doctor always taught me to use the best evidence-based medicine in practice. I took the traditional route of treating RA with non-steroidal anti-inflammatory drugs (NSAIDS, examples are ibuprofen, naproxen), steroids and methotrexate. Like Dr. Still's belief in the 1800's, I found the medicine's side effects more toxic to my body than the benefits and returned to my osteopathic philosophy to try to understand why my body became ill and why it developed this autoimmune disease. I decided to search for causes to try to find my health again. With the help of another osteopathic physician, I was able to look into causes such as poor nutrition, gastrointestinal tract (gut) health, stress, lack of rest and exercise. After becoming gluten free and researching nutrition to learn about anti-inflammatory foods, I made several dietary adjustments. I also looked at ways of reducing stress, staying active and getting the appropriate amount of sleep. I receive regular OMT treatments and have found acupuncture to also be very helpful. I am now off most of the RA medicines I had been taking, understand the triggers that cause my arthritis to flare and manage my disease, allowing me to enjoy my new found health.

Postgraduate Single Accreditation System in 2020

Can an MD learn osteopathy and do OMT? Yes! The MD (Accreditation Council of Graduate Medical Education or ACGME) and the DO (American Osteopathic Association or AOA) worlds came to a historical agreement at the level of graduate medical education. Due to an agreed single accreditation system, all AOA residency programs must obtain ACGME accreditation by 2020. After 2020, the plan is for all medical and surgical residency programs in the U.S. to be either ACGME accredited only, or ACGME with Osteopathic Recognition.

In the future, there will no longer be "AOA accredited only" programs or "dually accredited" programs (having both ACGME and AOA accreditation). The ACGME has specific requirements for a residency program to obtain osteopathic recognition and requires a separate application process. If medical students graduating from allopathic (MD) schools enter residency programs with osteopathic recognition and complete the program's requirements, they may practice OMT. Likewise, medical students graduating from osteopathic medical schools (DO) may do the same. For the DOs, choosing an ACGME residency with osteopathic recognition allows them to maintain and continue to improve their OMT skills.

This agreement *does not* affect medical schools, meaning a graduate of an osteopathic medical school is still a DO and a graduate of an allopathic medical school is still an MD.

A Day in the Life

As a board-certified Osteopathic Family Physician, I have had many practice options during my career. Originally, I started out in a traditional private practice. I delivered babies and took care of families of all ages from children to great grandparents. The only difference is I incorporated my osteopathic philosophy and OMT skills in their care. I always had an interest in teaching, so after I had my children, I was given the opportunity to enter academic medicine and graduate medical education. I currently spend some time during the week at a walk-in clinic at a large local university health center working as a family physician. I am also the Osteopathic Medical Director of Education at a Family and Internal Medicine Residency program at a large teaching hospital and I also teach medical bioethics at an allopathic medical school. A typical day for me may involve treating college students for various illnesses, seeing patients with resident physicians in training and medical students in our OMT clinic, practicing and teaching osteopathy and teaching students about different medical ethics issues. I also perform various administrative tasks that the ACGME requires for our hospital to maintain osteopathic recognition and lecture several times a month on all topics of osteopathy and family medicine.

Thus, you see a "typical" day in my life as an osteopathic physician isn't very typical at all and that's the advantage of becoming an osteopathic family physician. Many career options are available!

Career Outlook

According to U.S. News and World Report Best Jobs 2019, physicians which includes both Medical Doctors (MDs) and Doctors of Osteopathic Medicine (DOs) were ranked #9 in the 100 Best Jobs and #7 in Best Health Care Jobs and Best Paying Jobs. Physicians make a median salary of $208,000, with a 0.5% unemployment rate. There is an expected 7% employment growth for physicians between 2018 and 2028 with an estimated 55,400 new jobs available.

Search and Explore

American Academy of Family Practice
   http://www.aafp.org

American College of Osteopathic Family Physicians (ACOFP)
   http://www.acofp.org

I also recommend speaking to your own family doctor. There is nothing as valuable as having a role model or mentor to speak to in person, ask questions and obtain their personal perspective, as I did with my family physician. Look where it led me. That was a great resource when I was growing up!

Similar Jobs

Physician Assistant (PA)

Pharmacist

Podiatrist

Surgeon

CHAPTER 5

Registered Nurse

Eileen DeVries, BSN, RN, OCN, CBCN

Education:	Bachelor of Science in Nursing Degree	4 years
	OR	
	Associate's Degree in Nursing	2 years
	OR	
	Diploma in Nursing	2 years
License:	National Nursing Testing (NCLEX)/ License issued by State	
Median Income:	$71,730 (range, $50,800 - $106,530}	

Why I Became a Registered Nurse

At a young age, I was inspired by my mother who was a nurse, although like every other young girl I wanted to be a ballerina first. My mother would tell me stories about patients who were not feeling well and who miraculously got better. This was after the Visiting Nurse came to see them in their homes and made their booboos better. Obviously, this simplified view was child-like, but the nurse is focused on helping people become well. Throughout my childhood, I met many people who praised nurses (my Mom in particular) for being the person that carried them through bad events in their lives and helped them attain a better place. "You saved my life," was a common term I heard. I wanted to be that important to people.

Overview

Nurses affect people in so many different ways with the end result that the patients are able to care for themselves, and be healthier. A nurse is usually the medical professional for whom the patient spends the most time. The nurse is a teacher, a shoulder to cry on, a cheerleader and sometimes the bad guy or gal, all the while assessing the patient for improvement, worsening symptoms or life threatening emergencies. Nursing is one of the most respected professions, comprised of trust-worthy, ethical people. Nurses perform many technically difficult tasks, run complex machinery and constantly look forward to the next step in a patient's path to wellness. Nursing includes many specialties that are as varied as the parts of the body or in a variety of work environments.

If you think you are interested in nursing, volunteering in a hospital or nursing home can allow you to see the nursing profession in action. While in high school, a focus on math and sciences is helpful in preparing you for nursing school.

Specialties and Subspecialties

Obtaining certification in a specialty area of nursing can open many new roles in nursing. There are currently 183 certification specialties in nursing, everything from Critical Care, Forensics, Diabetes Management, Genetics and Oncology. Certification in a specialty can increase nursing job choices and salary. The venues for work in the field of nursing are quite varied and include hospitals seeing inpatients, or in the emergency department, or ambulatory settings (including emergency departments/clinics), outpatient clinics, long-term care facilities/nursing homes, private homes, government and community health agencies, urgent care centers, surgical centers, doctor's offices, schools, colleges, professional schools, sporting events/teams, hospice and palliative care services, managed care companies, in the OR, as well as corporate offices. There are even helicopter flight nurses, travelling nurses and nurses in war zones. Non-clinical RN occupations include: nurse educator, healthcare consultant, hospital administrator and nurse researcher. Nurses can find work in almost any environment.

Requirements

There are currently 1,973 accredited nursing schools in the U.S. conferring a Bachelor of Science in Nursing (BSN), an Associate's Degree (ADN) in nursing or a nursing diploma. Current requirements state that graduation from an accredited school and permission from the Board of Nursing in the state where you reside is required to be able to take the National Council Licensure Examination (NCLEX). Once a nurse has passed the NCLEX, the nursing candidate can start working as an RN. The average first time (of taking the examination) pass rate for RNs for the first quarter of 2019 was 86% (a total of 65,418 took the exam). Graduating high school and aspiring to be an RN, you can obtain a Bachelor of Science degree in nursing (BSN) in four years at a college or university. If you are already an RN, you can enroll in an RN-to-BSN program which is geared specifically for RNs who have an associate's degree in nursing (ADN) or nursing diploma. Going this route usually takes about two to three years.

Many of the same school course topics are taught in both the ADN and BSN programs. The four-year BSN program provides more in-depth knowledge and skills. As the field of nursing continues to become more competitive, more employers are requiring newly appointed RNs to hold a bachelor's degree. Some nursing coursework includes: Ethics, Anatomy and Physiology, Biochemistry, Statistics, Psychology, Patient Care, Biology, Introduction to Professional Nursing, and others.

Obtaining a job can be more difficult for an RN with an ADN or a nursing diploma. Most hospital organizations are moving to a minimal education requirement of a BSN for hiring. A nursing diploma is becoming less popular because it still takes two years to complete but does not confer a degree, unlike the ADN which provides a degree (after two years). Until the 1970's, these programs were one of the most common pathways to become a nurse. These diploma programs were the most traditional, long-standing form of healthcare education. Diploma programs were generally conferred by hospital-based nursing schools in the U.S. but are slowly being phasing out. These programs provide intensive hands-on training along with nursing coursework in areas such as Anatomy, Biology and Psychology. This experiential learning style provides students with basic nursing care knowledge. There are many online schools that provide transitional education to a BSN while you are working.

If you choose, you can obtain a master's degree in one and a half to two years. If you take this route, you can become more specialized as an Advanced Practice Registered Nurse (APRN). Some careers include: a Nurse Practitioner (NP), a Certified Nurse Midwife, a Clinical Nurse Specialist (CNS), a Certified Nurse Anesthetist (CRNA), a Clinical Nurse Leader (CNL), a Nurse Educator or a Nursing School Professor. Certified Nurse Anesthetist (see CRNA chapter) and NP are two of the more common advanced practitioner nursing specialties. NPs may order, perform and interpret diagnostic tests including laboratory data, electrocardiograms (EKGs) and X-rays (radiographs). APRNs may also prescribe medication, as a sole/independent practitioner. NP specialties include acute care, and psychiatry/mental health, primary care (pediatrics, adolescents, adults and adult gerontology), Women's Health (Obstetrics and Gynecology [OB/GYN]), and Neonatal and Emergency certifications. Nurse Practitioners, with more advanced training, can practice in subspecialty areas such as Medical/Surgical areas, Cardiology, Renal/Urology, Perinatal Care, Long-Term Care, Orthopedics, Rehabilitation medicine, Pulmonary medicine, Pediatrics, Gerontology, Emergency department/Trauma, Post-Partum care, Psychiatry, Critical Care, Dermatology, Hospice, Oncology and Public Health. Surgical NPs can perform minor surgical procedures or assist in major surgical procedures. Nurse Practitioners often are on college and university campuses working in (or running) Health Services. NPs can also have their own private practices, as well as work in any of the settings where RNs would work.

A Day in the Life of a Registered Nurse

My day as an outpatient oncology nurse begins by reviewing the patient schedule. I must review the chemotherapy plan for the patient, ensure that we are ordering the appropriate blood work and that all necessary X-rays (such as echocardiograms which are necessary to assure heart health or chest radiographs to assure proper catheter placement) are available to administer those drugs. If these are not in place, then it will be necessary for me to contact the doctor to ensure that we obtain the correct orders or tests prior to treatment. When the patient arrives, my assessment starts. I begin with just a visual of the patient...as he or she walks to the treatment chair: is he or she walking normally without pain? Is he or she breathing easily or do they appear nervous? I obtain basic vital signs, such as blood pressure, pulse, temperature and weight and then ask the patient how he or she is feeling. This helps to provide the starting tasks. For most patients receiving cancer chemotherapy (cancer fighting drugs), I must establish an IV access line into their vein so that I can obtain laboratory values (also see Phlebotomist chapter). After I send the tests to the laboratory and the results are back, the medical team evaluates them to ensure that the patient meets the treatment parameters. I then calculate the chemotherapy dose to ensure that the physician has calculated the dose correctly and that we have selected the correct drug for that particular patient's cancer type (a pharmacist also checks that the dose is correct for any particular patient, after the medical team orders the drug). Each time I see a patient for treatment, I listen to what he or she says about the treatment and the side effects. I am constantly assessing what patients have learned about the procedure since every conversation is an opportunity to teach them more about the disease or reinforce their actions as a way to improve their health. I administer medications to prevent treatment side effects (these are called pre-medications) and then I start the chemotherapy treatment. Many of the available chemotherapy drugs are dangerous. Cancer chemotherapy drugs require safe handling and special precautions to avoid potential harm to the people around the patient: the family and the nurses who administer the medications and the pharmacists who prepare the medication. Educating the patients and their caregivers is part of every conversation. After the chemotherapy is completed, I remove the IV and the patient goes home. My perception is that there are so many people who are afraid of cancer and its treatment. Because of this, patients often do not hear the necessary information they need for them to do well during their treatment(s). As their nurse, it is my responsibility to reinforce the information they need and not overwhelm them. As a nurse, you must be willing to repeat yourself until it clicks for each patient!

One of my best memories of patients is the story of Cathy C (I have changed the name for privacy). Cathy C was diagnosed with breast cancer and needed chemotherapy for five months. She was afraid that she would not be able to be a Mom to her children. She came for treatment crying and cried throughout the treatment. She cried every time she came for the first three treatments. The Saturday after her third treatment, Mark and Tom (her children), each had a ballgame. She went to both games and did everything a Mom does and she did not get sick or miss anything. When treatment number four arrived, Cathy walks in through the door smiling and laughing. I was totally shocked and asked Cathy, "What is going on?" She said, "This is only chemotherapy and I can do anything I need to for my family. I don't know why I was so upset." Tom and Mark, having two different ballgames on one day, finally helped Cathy realize that she could manage chemotherapy and still be a happy and healthy Mom to her two boys. Cathy completed her chemotherapy and went to every event Mark and Tom had during treatment cycle without missing a beat. That's the joy of being a nurse.

Career Outlook

U.S. News and World Report ranks the career of RN as #15 in the 100 Best jobs, and #19 in Best Health Care jobs. The Bureau of Labor Statistics projects 12% employment growth for RNs through 2028, with an estimated 371,500 jobs opening. RNs have about a 1.4% unemployment rate. In 2018, RNs made a median salary of $71,730, while the best paid 25% made $85,960 in that year, the lowest-paid 25% made $57,340.

U.S. News and World Report ranks the career of NP as #7 in the 100 Best Jobs, and #5 in Best Health Care Jobs. NPs are well paid, with the top 50% of nurse practitioners bringing home six-figure salaries, with a low unemployment rate of 1.1%. The Bureau of Labor Statistics projects 28% percent employment growth between 2018 and 2028, with about 53,300 new jobs. The median salary of NPs in 2018 was $107,030, with the best-paid 25% making $123,070, and the lowest-paid 25% having made $88,810.

U.S. News and World Report ranks the career of Nurse Midwives as #16 in the 100 Best jobs, and #14 in Best Health Care jobs. The Bureau of Labor Statistics projects 16% employment growth for Midwifery through 2028, as Midwifery is a rapidly growing field of practice, with an estimated 1,000 jobs opening through 2028. There are many areas of the country that are medically underserved or are not served at all by maternity care providers. Nurse midwives are advanced practice registered nurses (APRNs) who see women of all ages for annual exams, regular pregnancy exams, menopausal care and more. Nurse midwives can handle normal pregnancies, but only an obstetrician and gynecologist (physician) can perform a cesarean section or more complicated pregnancies and procedures. In 2018, the median salary for Nurse Midwives was $103,770. The best-paid 25% made $120,830, while the lowest-paid 25% made $86,570.

Search and Explore

Oncology Nursing Certification Corporation
   https://www.oncc.org/certifications/certified-breast-care-nurse-cbcn

American Nursing Association (ANA)
   http://www.nursingworld.org

American Association of Nurse Practitioners (AANP)
   http://www.aanp.org

Oncology Nursing Society
   https://www.ons.org

Travel Nursing: An Overview
   https://www.nursejournal.org/travel-nursing/traveling-nursing-an-overview/

U.S. News and World Report Best Jobs 2019 Nursing Aide Salary
   https://money.usnews.com/careers/best-jobs/nursing-aide/salary

Stokowski LA. APRN Prescribing Law: A State-by-State Summary Published January 4, 2018
   https://www.medscape.com/viewarticle/440315

Case Management Society of America
   http://www.cmsa.org

American College Health Association
   https://www.acha.org/

Similar Occupations

Nurse Practitioner (NP)

Certified Registered Nurse Anesthetist (CRNA) - see chapter on CRNA

Doctor of Nursing (ND) - further education (doctorate)

Licensed Practical Nurses (LPNs) or Licensed Vocational Nurses (LVNs) - work under RNs and doctors. One-year of school and license required. Median pay $46,240 (2018)

Nursing Assistant - train between four and 12 weeks

Certified Nurses Aide (CNA) - high school diploma/GED plus nursing assistant training which are provided by community colleges, trade schools and medical facilities. Make sure you enroll in a program that is approved by your state's nursing board. In 2018, Nurses Aides made $28,540 (range, $21,290 - $39,560).

Patient Care Assistants or Patient Transport - transport patients and clean treatment areas - High school diploma/GED

CHAPTER 6

Certified Registered Nurse Anesthetist (CRNA)

Michael Greco, PhD, DNP, CRNA

Education:	Bachelor's in Nursing Degree	4 years
	Clinical Experience	Minimum 1-year critical care nursing experience as an RN
	CRNA training Program	2.5 - 3 years*
License:	Registered Professional Nurse or Advanced Practice Registered Nurse (Depending on state practicing Nurse Anesthesia)	
Certification:	National Board of Certification and Recertification for Nurse Anesthetists (NBCRNA)	
Median income:	$167,950 (range, $116,820 - $208,000)	

As of 2020, All CRNA programs will be at the doctorate level issuing a Doctor of Nursing Practice Degree.

Why I Became a Certified Nurse Anesthetist

As a critical care nurse educator working in a demanding New York City trauma center, I was always intrigued with the advanced knowledge and skill-set of Certified Registered Nurse Anesthetists (CRNAs) whenever we interacted professionally. Whenever the CRNAs were endorsing their patients to the critical care registered nurse (RN) after surgery in the Surgical Intensive Care unit (SICU), I would witness their demeanor as they projected and exuded a high level of professionalism and confidence. They comprehensively managed their patients with pain control, hemodynamic stability and advanced airway support. The nurse anesthetists noticed my enthusiasm toward their role and educated me about their practice in both the OR, remote locations throughout the hospital and obstetrical unit. I was very attracted to the high degree of autonomy and professional respect the CRNAs commanded. They carried a heavy load of responsibility and were respected by the entire healthcare team. Their compassion, vigilance in their responsibilities and advocacy toward their patients engaged me and led me to further research this career.

I have been a nurse since 1994, and have worked in different settings including: critical care; emergency room; post-anesthesia care/recovery unit (PACU); occupational health (for American Airlines); and in nursing staff education, before I embarked on the nurse anesthesia profession. As these opportunities arose, I was always taking risks. I learned that one could not accomplish anything good without being adventuresome. Nobody was going to offer an opportunity to me without me being a little daring. That can be simply changing jobs from medical center to medical center, to simply changing nursing specialties. After taking that leap and moving to nurse anesthesia, I look back and think that I would not be so developed in this noble profession without any risk taking. I left my full time RN job, was commissioned in the U.S. Army and enrolled in CRNA school full-time.

I found the field of anesthesia appealing as a specialty since one can practice it in many different settings/locations. Some locations include hospitals, military establishments, outpatient ambulatory surgery centers, trauma centers, obstetrical centers and rural areas, where CRNAs are often the sole anesthesia provider. While enrolled in my CRNA program, I decided to commission in the U.S. Army Reserves. During my CRNA training, I practiced in a busy trauma center in Brooklyn, New York, on a full-time basis. This made employment difficult. The U.S. Army had many financial incentives and stipends, of which I took advantage while I was in school. This really helped offset the cost of my CRNA education and allowed me to have additional spending money, so I could give 100% to my career, without worrying about finances.

After graduating from the SUNY Downstate Brooklyn Nurse Anesthesia program with my master's degree in 2001, I practiced in a large medical center in Manhattan and was privileged to care for a diverse patient population. After graduating, I served in the U.S. Army reserves for eight years and had the honor and privilege to care for our nation's soldiers and their families as well as veterans who have fought for our great country.

In 2005-2010, I was deployed in the U.S. Army as a nurse anesthetist and had the opportunity to serve in Germany, Italy, Iraq and many other army bases located thought the continental U.S. This experience was one I will cherish and value for the rest of my life. I worked in many different practice settings. I was exposed to, and was challenged, with limited available resources in places like Iraq. Most of the anesthesia departments where I practiced during my military career were "all CRNA" teams. Standards of care were held high by all CRNA department heads and quality care was always provided. In 2010, I graduated with my Doctor of Nurse Practice degree from the University of Alabama. Since this time, I have been teaching and sharing my CRNA experience and knowledge with the next generation of nurse anesthetists at Columbia University in New York. I recently attained my PhD in nursing and have graduated as a nurse scientist. I hope to generate and develop new scientific knowledge for nurse anesthesia, which will help to move healthcare and the profession forward. I currently serve as the Director of Nurse Anesthesia Services for Northwell Health in New York.

Choosing a profession as a CRNA can be both extremely rewarding and difficult, since you help patients under ordinary and extraordinary circumstances. Patients inspire you during days you may struggle – they help you through challenging days! Becoming a CRNA is a long, demanding journey, but when you get to the end, you will look back and recognize that it was worth all the sacrifices.

Overview

Nurse anesthetists, the first healthcare providers committed to the specialty of anesthesia, have their roots in the 1800s, when nurses first gave anesthesia to injured warriors on the battlefield during the Civil War. The CRNA credential came into existence in 1956. CRNAs provide anesthesia in collaboration with surgeons, anesthesiologists, dentists, podiatrists and other qualified healthcare professionals. When a nurse anesthetist administers anesthesia, the medical profession recognizes it as the practice of nursing. When an anesthesiologist administers anesthesia, the medical profession recognizes it as the practice of medicine. Regardless of whether the anesthesia administration educational background is in nursing or medicine, all anesthesia professionals administer anesthesia under the same principles. Nurse anesthetists have been providing anesthesia care to patients in the U.S. for more than 150 years. According to the American Association of Nurse Anesthetists (AANA) 2016 Practice Profile Survey, CRNAs are anesthesia professionals who safely administer *approximately 43 million anesthetics* to patients in the U.S. each year. CRNAs are the primary providers of anesthesia care in rural America, enabling healthcare facilities in these medically underserved areas to offer obstetrical, surgical, pain management and trauma stabilization services. In some states, CRNAs are the sole anesthesia providers in nearly 100% of the rural hospitals. Today, more than 48,000 CRNAs and student registered nurse anesthetists (SRNAs) administer more than 34 million anesthetics to patients in all 50 states each year. CRNAs collaborate with other members of the patient care team including surgeons, radiologists, cardiologists, gastroenterologists, podiatrists, obstetricians, anesthesiologists, nurses, technicians, other physician specialists and OR personnel. CRNAs are responsible for their patients' safety and comfort throughout the procedure, monitoring vital signs (e.g., blood pressure, heart rate and respiration), and adjusting the depth of anesthesia as necessary. In addition, CRNAs are always prepared to analyze situations and respond quickly to all patients' needs, especially in emergencies.

Specialties and Subspecialties

In collaboration with the AANA, Middle Tennessee School of Nurse Anesthesia provides CRNAs with the potential to complete a 12-month post-graduate fellowship in pain management. Two different programs are currently available, one in advanced pain management, and one in acute surgical pain management. This fellowship incorporates evidence-based knowledge to provide a clinically oriented multidisciplinary training environment for CRNA students to study comprehensive pain management. Visit: https://www.aana.com/ce-education/ pain-management/advanced-pain-management-fellowship-program for more information on these programs since the requirements continue to change.

Requirements

To qualify as a Nurse Anesthetist, you must have a bachelor's degree in nursing (or other appropriate bachelor's degree); Registered Nurse licensure in the U.S., its territories or protectorates; a minimum of one-year critical care practice as a registered nurse; and the successful completion of both an accredited nurse anesthesia educational program and the national certification examination.

The AANA and Council on Accreditation (COA) requires applicants who matriculate into nurse anesthesia programs to have completed at least one year (365 days) of critical care experience as an RN. One must obtain this Intensive Care Unit (ICU) experience in a critical care area within the U.S., its territories or a U.S. military hospital outside of the States. During this experience, the RN needs to have developed critical decision-making and psychomotor skills, competency in patient assessment and the ability to use and interpret advanced monitoring techniques. The COA defines critical care areas as one where, on a routine basis, the RN manages one or more of the following: invasive hemodynamic monitors (such as pulmonary artery catheter, CVP [central venous pressure], arterial); cardiac assist devices; mechanical ventilation and vasoactive infusions. Examples of critical care units may include but are not limited to: SICU, Cardiothoracic ICU, Cardiac Care Unit (CCU), Medical ICU, Neurology or Neurosurgical Intensive Care Unit, Burn-Trauma ICU and Pediatric Intensive Care Unit.

In addition to the above general requirements, individual programs have specific admission criteria required for their specific academic institutions. You can find a complete list of nurse anesthesia programs and information specific to each individual program at the Council on Accreditation of Nurse Anesthesia Educational Programs Website (see References). CRNA recertification is every four years.

A Day in the Life of a CRNA

A typical day in the life of a CRNA starts very early. My alarm sounds at 5:30 am and I leave home and head to the hospital by 6:30 am. One advantage I have is that the hospital where I practice is 20 minutes away from where I live. For my colleagues who travel a further distance to get to work, their day starts much earlier than mine. I shower, eat breakfast and prepare my lunch and snacks to take to work. Since CRNAs generally have only a 30 minute lunch break and the timing is inconsistent, the hospital cafeteria may be closed. To play it safe, I bring my lunch as a security knowing a noon lunch break is not guaranteed. Once arriving at work, I head straight for the locker room. The locker room is where all surgical staff including doctors, nurses, scrub techs and anesthesia providers change from their street clothes worn to and from home, to the surgical attire known as scrubs. Medical personnel wear scrubs in the OR for many reasons. Scrubs help OR personnel identify contaminants such as bodily fluids. Scrubs are economical to replace. They are laundered using harsh chemicals and high temperatures killing disease and non-disease causing microorganisms, and they protect personal clothing from damage. The next step I complete before I can enter the OR is to place blue shoe covers known as booties over my shoes. We wear these booties to prevent dirt, dust or even bacteria on our shoes from scattering around the OR, potentially infecting the surgical patient. After changing into scrubs and putting on my booties, I put a surgical cap on my head (all of this is collectively called "donning surgical garb"). The reason we wear surgical caps on our heads is to prevent hair from falling into the sterile surgical field. A small piece of hair can cause a severe infection for a patient. Once I am fully dressed in my proper OR attire, I enter the OR and check my assignment. This is a list that tells me in what surgical suite I will be working, with whom I will be working (e.g., staff, surgeons) and the surgical procedures I will be performing. As a CRNA, we are trained to anesthetize patients during all sorts of surgical cases from simple finger surgeries to complex open-heart surgeries. This is why I must check my assignment, so I know what equipment, medications and supplies I will need for the day. As I enter the room, I go to the head of the OR bed which is referred to as the OR table and check that the table is functioning without any apparent problems. I would not want my patient sleeping on a bed and then we realize it is broken. Next, I perform a safety check on my anesthesia machine. The anesthesia workstation is a large piece of equipment we use in the OR to deliver the anesthetic gases to the patient. This machine has a breathing machine on it to help patients breathe during surgery, six special gases to choose from that we deliver to the patient and advanced monitoring technology so I can observe and monitor the heart rhythm, oxygenation, blood pressure, temperature and other patient vital signs during the surgery. I draw up all necessary medications, set-up IV infusions, and gather any other essential supplies.

I then head to the area where patients are waiting for surgery, as the preoperative nurse prepares them. I introduce myself to the patient and take a comprehensive medical history and perform a physical exam. I look at the patient's chart and assess all laboratory data and any preoperative testing that may have been performed such as electrocardiograms (ECGs) and breathing tests. From this information, I develop a safe anesthetic plan for my patient. This plan includes what drugs I will use and how much I will use, what tubes I will need, what anesthetic I will administer and any special precautions that I will need to take. I also explain all risks and benefits of the anesthesia to the patient and describe his or her expected anesthetic course. This interaction usually makes the patient and his or her family feel much more comfortable and relaxed. I obtain consent from the patient to receive anesthesia. Consent is the patient's permission for me to administer the prescribed anesthesia. Since I practice in a team model, I then call my anesthesiologist, who is assigned to my room, and about three other CRNA rooms and present the patient and discuss my anesthetic plan. Presenting the patient means I tell the anesthesiologist all about the patient, his or her medical history, medical problems and what surgery he or she is having that day. Once we agree on the plan and the OR is ready, I bring the patient into the surgical suite.

Once we arrive in the OR suite, I introduce the patient to the surgical team and then lay him or her down on the OR table. I start the IV in his or her arm so I can start administering medication, which will relax the patient. I place the patient on all the monitors (e.g., the heart monitor, the oxygen monitor and the blood pressure cuff) and begin giving him or her a mask with flowing oxygen. I ask the patient to take a deep breath and simultaneously administer IV medication that puts him or her to sleep. This part of the anesthetic course is called the induction. Unfortunately, it is not just one medication that patients receive, but rather four to six different medications that work together to ensure that the patient is sleeping and comfortable. This helps the patient feel no pain when the surgeon makes the surgical incision. This is a critical part of my job, which is also a dangerous period for the patient. Considerable concentration and focus is necessary when inducing a patient. Once the patient is sleeping, I place a breathing tube in his or her windpipe. This is so I can deliver gases into the lungs, which then enter the blood and then to the brain. This is to keep the patient sleeping during the surgery. I take the tube out before the patient wakes up. The only way the patient may know the tube was there is if he or she complains about a sore throat or throat dryness in the 24 hours after surgery.

After the induction, the OR team preps the patient and covers him or her with sterile sheets. During this time, I monitor the patient very closely making sure I am delivering the correct amount of anesthesia keeping the patient safe and comfortable as promised. I may need to inject more medicine in the IV or increase or decrease the gas flow depending on the patient's response. If the patient loses a considerable amount of blood, it is my job to replace the blood and administer a transfusion. If the surgeon needs the OR table adjusted, it is the CRNAs job to adjust that accordingly, as well.

Once the surgical procedure is over, I begin waking up my patient. I need to ensure the patient is breathing normally, and that he or she is able to regain all muscle strength before I remove the breathing tube. This part of the surgery is called the emergence and is also a critical time for the patient. Once the patient meets a specific criterion, I remove the breathing tube and replace it with an oxygen mask. I wait a few minutes then call for a portable bed called a stretcher. Transport workers then deliver the patient to the PACU where another nurse cares for the patient and monitors him or her during the immediate recovery from surgery and the anesthesia. I give the nurse report (this means, telling workers in the PACU about the patient history), and telling the patient all the events that transpired during the surgery. I also list and report all medications that I used during the procedure. I make sure the patient is stable and pain free before I leave the PACU to head back to the OR. I then reset my room for the next scheduled patient.

Career Outlook

According to U.S. News and World Report, a Nurse Anesthetist is ranked #3 in Best Health Care Jobs, #5 in 100 Best Jobs, and #11 in Best Paying Jobs. The median salary is $167,950, with an unemployment rate of 0.4%. According to the Bureau of Labor Statistics, the profession will grow by about 17% by the year 2028, translating into 7,600 new job openings.

Search and Explore

The American Association of Nurse Anesthetists
  http://www.aana.com

Council on Accreditation of Nurse Anesthesia Educational Programs
  http://home.coa.us.com/

Nurse Anesthetist Programs
  https://www.registerednursing.org/nurse-anesthetist/programs/

Santiago AC. States That Allow CRNAs to Practice Without Physician Supervision
  Published May 8, 2019

  https://www.verywellhealth.com/which-states-allow-crnas-to-practice-independently-1736102

Similar Careers

Registered Nurse (RN) - Bachelor's Degree

Surgical Technologist

CHAPTER 7

Case Manager

Anne Llewellyn, RN-BC, MS, BHSA, CCM, and CRRN

Education:	Bachelor's Degree	4 years
License:	Nursing or Social Work*	
Meanian Salary:	$77,877 (range, $71,180 and $85,301)**	

Social workers, respiratory therapists, physical therapists and pharmacists can also be case managers, so the degree and licensure would differ depending on the field of study.

** *Salaries are dependent upon a variety of factors including job location*

Why I Became a Nurse Case Manager

I became a case manager when I moved to Florida in 1988 after being a critical care nurse for most of my career. I learned about case management through a friend who had just moved into this role. She explained her job and I found it very interesting. She told me the company she worked for was looking for nurses in South Florida where I was living. I called the contact she gave me and asked for an application. I filled out the application and mailed it. A few days later I received a call to come in for an interview. I was a little nervous since I did not know much about case management but wanted to learn more, so I decided to go. In 1988, there was no 'google' so I had nowhere to really learn about a case manager's role. I also did not know how to prepare for the interview other than what my friend had told me.

I went for the interview and met the Supervisor of the Case Management (CM) Department. She asked me several questions about what I did as a nurse in my current role as an Emergency Room nurse. She also asked what I had done in my career prior to moving to Florida and what I knew about CM. I told her I did not know anything, except what my friend told me. She explained to me that CM was a field that many nurses moved into because they were able to look at the patient from a holistic view and had clinical knowledge to understand the complex medical conditions to which patients presented. In addition, Case Managers (CMs) were aware of complications that might occur in patients since they generally understood or could learn about the conditions due to their background clinical knowledge. She said nurses were good communicators and organized, and could troubleshoot problems which are key strategies of effective CM. She ended with saying that in her view, CM boils down to providing good nursing care since CMs were in place to see that the patient had a voice, was listened to and had the resources to meet his or her individual needs.

CMs help patients understand their diagnosis and how to best care for themselves once they are stable. It is important that patient care is based on evidence, is performed in a timely manner, and is in the least restrictive environment, for the most affordable price. One main CM goal is to help conserve healthcare dollars when someone is sick or injured.

The person who interviewed me explained that this job would focus on patients who had suffered catastrophic illnesses such as spinal cord injuries, head injuries and organ transplants. As a nurse CM, my role would be to meet with the patient and work with the medical team to coordinate patient care throughout one's healthcare journey.

At this interview, I liked what I heard and felt I could use my skills as a critical care nurse to be an effective CM. The Supervisor offered me the job and I accepted. Since I was new, I underwent training and was assigned to another nurse CM who served as my mentor.

Overview

A CMs purpose is to help contain costs for those who are sick or injured. The medical profession views CMs as advanced practice professionals, meaning they enter the CM practice after a few years of clinical experience. Nurses are the largest professional group that work as CMs. Case Management is a multidisciplinary field, so professionals other than nurses work as professional case managers, including: social workers, respiratory therapists, physical therapists, pharmacists and others who have expertise in specific areas. The most important part of case management for each professional is to work within their scope of practice. Working as a CM provides autonomy and allows each professional to optimally utilize his or her skills. Finding the area of practice is important. Finding your optimal workplace or patient setting is the key to your success. Nurse case managers handle complex patient assignments. The case manager would call a patient to help him or her navigate the healthcare system so he or she can receive the care that he or she requires in an efficient manner. Basically, the nurse CMs role is to educate and empower patients, so they can care and advocate for themselves. Case managers help patients (and their caregivers) to understand their diagnosis, their care plan and ensure they have the necessary tools and resources to meet their needs.

You can apply the Pareto Business Principle to medicine and provide the justification for Case Management. It basically states that in the U.S. we spend 80% of the healthcare dollars on 20% of the population. With healthcare costs increasing in the trillions of dollars range, having a CM to work with high-risk, high-cost patients, and with the patient's healthcare team to coordinate evidence-based care that is safe and cost effective, makes total sense.

Specialties and Subspecialties

CMs can be found in every sector of the healthcare system. These individuals may be working in the hospital as a pediatric nurse CM or working in a skilled care or nursing facility specializing in geriatrics. Another role is as a telephonic nurse CM. Most of these roles are in a managed care or insurance company. Some nurse case managers also work in workers compensation. These CMs work with injured workers to ensure they receive the medical care that will help them return to work. Case management spans the human life span. Nurse case managers can work with high risk mothers when they are pregnant, they can work with children of all ages, and they can work with adults, including the elderly, so there are many different opportunities. Following are some different CM practice settings to consider:

Hospital Case Manager: These CMs work with patients who have complex problems. There are usually several physicians working with the patient, so it is important that patient care is coordinated so that all providers know what each other is doing, and all are working toward a common goal. Often, a pharmacist is also part of the team he or she can ensure the patient is on the right medications, is not experiencing any adverse medication effects (e.g., drug reaction, drug interaction; see glossary), is on the appropriate dose, and is appropriately monitored for the best outcome. Additionally, sometimes a healthcare practitioner decreases or increases a patient's medications (e.g., on fewer medications) to improve his or her care. Once a patient is ready to leave the hospital, the case manager may need to order equipment or resources. The CM helps the patient safely and effectively transition to the next care setting.

Managed Care Case Manager: These CMs work directly for the Managed Care or insurance company to assist their patient-members to manage complex medical problems, including following them after a severe accident/injury. CMs can also work on the prevention side to help people change behavior so they can lose weight, stop smoking or address a drug or alcohol problem. Most managed care CMs work telephonically. To work telephonically, you need to have good phone assessment skills. Good listening skills and the ability to build a relationship are important competencies you must have to be successful in this role.

Pediatric Case Management: This CM works with children of all ages when they are sick or injured. In addition to the child, the CM also works with child's parent(s) or guardian(s) as well as teachers in the school system. The pediatric CM educates and provides support for the patient and his or her families. Helping children learn how to care for themselves and recover the best they can is important, since many of these conditions can be life-long challenges.

Workers Compensation: When someone is injured on the job, he or she is covered under their employer's workers compensation policy instead of his or her own health insurance. When injured, a person may not be able to work, which can be costly to the employer and the employee. Having a Workers Compensation CM in place to ensure the injured workers receive the care they need to return to work is important.

Military: Case Managers work in the military healthcare system as well as the VA to help the service members recover from an injury or illness sustained by working in the military.

Requirements

There are a few ways one can become a CM. Nurses become CMs after they have a few years of nursing practice. The requirements for those who want to become a CM are to have 2-3 years of healthcare experience. Having this foundation helps the CM think outside the box, communicate effectively, build relationships and affect change. Case management strives to be proactive and to anticipate issues that might arise and to offer solutions to avoid those setbacks. These skills are important for professionals who enter the field. Other professionals, like pharmacists, can become case managers, but the training is not as well defined. Usually after a few years of experience in working with patients in managed care, or in a specialty pharmacy or MTM, pharmacists become CMs. However, most do not follow in the certification path that nurses do through the Case Management Society of American (CMSA).

Case managers are an added layer to the healthcare system, so it is important for those who work as CMs to have a way to demonstrate their value. Their value would be evident by showing the work they do in making a difference to contain healthcare costs, improve access to care and ensure safe, quality care.

The CMSA has developed the Case Management Standards of Practice. In addition, once a nurse case manager has a few years of experience, he or she can become certified. To become a certified CM you need twelve months of acceptable full-time case management employment experience in the last five years, and supervision by a board-certified case manager (CCM). Your

Supervisor must also be certified for at least one year at the time of your application. Certification allows a case management professional to validate the expertise he or she has in the field. Having a CCM (Certified Case Manager) also offers the consumer a way to know that their CM is qualified and meets a standard set by the certification body. In order to become certified as a CM you need to have a qualifying education which can be either: (1) a license to practice; (2) a Bachelor's degree or Master's degree from an institution in a Health or Human Services Field; or (3) a certification from a list of related practices; and fulfill an employment category, either: (1) twelve months of full-time case management experience supervised by a CCM; (2) twenty-four months full-time CM experience, where your supervisor does not need to be a CCM; or (3) twelve months full-time CM experience as a Supervisor of individuals who provide case management (meeting certain criteria which the CCM certification guide defines).

A Day in the Life of a Case Manager

Other case managers may have a different story since many of us have different experiences. This is my story. I worked as a catastrophic CM when I entered the practice. I was able to work from home. Working at home sounds attractive but it requires one to be disciplined and organized. My day would start by checking my work email since I would receive new patient cases this way. I would also receive emails about my current patient caseload.

Most days I would have appointments where I had to meet a new patient, visit an existing patient in the hospital or attend a staff conference with a patient in a rehabilitation hospital. Sometimes I would meet a patient and his or her caregiver in his or her home or at the doctor's office. I would prepare for that meeting by reviewing the patient's file/chart so I knew what I had to do. This way, I could be as efficient as possible. I would make a list of questions and determine with whom I had to meet. I would give myself enough time to arrive at appointments on time. Planning and organizing are important skills CMs must have. In addition, I would reply to any necessary phone calls, or make calls to check on the patients I was following. Daily, I would provide updates, review my cases and share my strategies and care plans with my supervisor. My supervisor would offer helpful suggestions in managing my patients. I was always the patient's advocate and was in contact with the care team. CMs also know the patient's health benefit plan since they are in contact with the insurance company. My goal was to keep one step ahead, so I could offer solutions and ideas that would streamline my patient's care, and ensure it was meeting their needs. Close patient monitoring would allow me to be aware of any imminent issues, so I could notify the healthcare team, and modify and quickly resolve care plans, if needed.

Search and Explore

American Case Management Association
   http://www.acmaweb.org

Case Management Society of America and Standards of Practice
   http://www.cmsa.org/
   http://www.cmsa.org/sop

Commission for Case Manager Certification
   https://ccmcertification.org

CMSA Today Providing insight from CM leaders in practice. Published 2016
   http://www.nxtbook.com/naylor/CMSQ/CMSQ0316/index.php#/0

RN Case Manager Salary and Job Outlook Published 2018
   http://nursejournal.org/nursing-case-management/rn-case-manager-salary-and-job-outlook/

Social Community for Nurses Worldwide
   https://nursejournal.org/

Similar Careers

Social Worker

Registered Nurse

Psychologist

CHAPTER 8

Physician Assistant

Julie Gruber, PA-C, MPAS

Education:	Bachelor's Degree	4 years
	PA Degree	2-3 years
	Residency	1 year
Certification/ License:	Physician Assistant National Certifying Examination (PANCE)	
Median income:	$108,610 (range, $65,620-$142,210)	

Why I Became a Physician Assistant

Growing up, I was surrounded by physicians and medical practitioners. Both my mom and grandfather were medical doctors and encouraged me to pursue a career in medicine. I was fascinated by all the illustrations in their medical books and the fascinating cases they discussed. For me it was almost innate to pursue a career in medicine. I never considered anything else. In high school I was in the medical science program, and in college I majored in biology, gearing up to apply to medical school. When I was completing my undergraduate degree, people did not understand or appreciate the Physician Assistant (PA) profession as it is today, so I never considered it. I don't think I knew the specifics of the role. I was beginning to consider applying to medical school, when one of my closest friends enrolled in PA school. When she applied to PA school, she offered her advice. Following our conversation, I was on a quest to figure out about a career as a PA. That same day I researched the PA profession, then I applied to the program. I met all the requirements since I had been working in an ophthalmologist's office during college and had more than the required direct patient contact hours. Later that year, I was fortunate enough to receive an interview invitation and was later accepted to start in August 2010. Despite a challenging three years of education and clinical rotations, acceptance into the PA program was analogous to me winning the lottery. It was a gateway to me becoming a medical provider, working with an amazing team, and loving my job every day, all while giving me the flexibility to have an outstanding quality of life.

Overview

Physician Assistants are healthcare providers who work together as a team with a supervising physician to provide diagnostic and therapeutic care to patients. PAs obtain and review patient's medical histories, examine patients, order and interpret diagnostic tests, provide treatment, prescribe medications and educate and counsel patients.

Physician Assistants work in all medical specialties, including primary care, family medicine, internal medicine, obstetrics and gynecology and emergency medicine. PAs may also work in general surgery, in surgical subspecialties, in long term care facilities and provide visits to patients who are unable to leave their homes. Many PAs have the time and flexibility to work in more than one subspecialty.

Preparing to become a PA can start as early as high school. Students may consider volunteering in a healthcare setting to gain patient contact experience and learn as much as they can about the profession. Students also should enroll in science classes to build a strong foundation for beginning undergraduate education as they pursue a career as a PA.

Specialties and Subspecialties

PAs can specialize in family/internal medicine, pediatrics, obstetrics and gynecology, surgery, surgical subspecialties, critical care, cardiology, orthopedics and psychiatry to name a few. The National Commission on Certification of Physician Assistants (NCPA) now offers recognition for certain specialties by offering PAs to take a Certification of Added Qualifications (CAQ) exam, once they have met specific prerequisites based on experience within their specialty. Seven CAQ specialties exist at the time of this writing. They include: cardiovascular and thoracic surgery, emergency medicine, hospital medicine, orthopedic surgery, nephrology, pediatrics and psychiatry.

Requirements

To be admitted into a PA program, you must fulfill certain prerequisite class requirements which you usually achieve through a four year bachelor's degree program. Required classes include the basic sciences such as chemistry, biology, microbiology, anatomy and physiology. All programs have specific requirements which vary but overall, individuals who apply must have healthcare work experience or have accrued a specific amount of "hands on" patient care. Many programs now require prospective students to take the Graduate Record Exam (GRE). All programs require selected applicants to undergo an interview process prior to admission.

At present, there are 243 PA programs in the U.S. which the Accreditation Review Commission on Education for the Physician Assistant (ARC-PA) accredits. ARC-PA defines the standards of the PA profession and education, evaluating programs to comply with these standards.

All PA programs are at least 26 months long and can be completed within three academic years. The program includes didactic (classroom) and clinical (seeing patients) phases. In the classroom, PA students study advanced sciences including: anatomy, physiology, biochemistry, pharmacology, pathophysiology and behavioral sciences. The clinical phase requires PA students to complete at least 2000 hours of clinical rotations in family and internal medicine, obstetrics and gynecology, emergency medicine, pediatrics and general surgery. Students must also complete several elective rotations of their choice. Some electives include critical care medicine, surgery or any interest area. Upon successful completion of all classes, the program awards graduates with a master's degree.

Once PAs graduate from an accredited program they are eligible to apply for their medical license. This requires passing the Physician Assistant National Certification Exam (PANCE), administered by the NCCPA. All states have different licensing requirements, but once you pass the PANCE, you can apply for a license in any U.S. state.

To maintain certification as a PA, an individual must complete 100 CME hours every two years. PAs must also pay a certification maintenance fee to NCCPA every two years, a licensing fee every three years and pass the Physician Assistant National Recertifying Exam (PANRE) every ten years.

A Day in the Life of a PA

As a critical care PA, my day begins at 7 a.m. when I start to take care of my critically ill patients in our hospital. I receive a report (a review of the patients during the last shift) from the overnight PA about any new patients admitted, and any relevant happenings of my patients from overnight. I am then able to review any laboratory test results from the prior day/night, review any imaging study results such as radiographs (X-rays) or CT scans and review any treatment plan updates that the overnight healthcare team made. Next, I examine all my patients, review their medications and current medical orders. With all the information I have gathered, I am now prepared for interdisciplinary team rounds with the intensive care attending physician, nurse, pharmacist, physical therapist and any other members of the healthcare team taking care of my patient. I present my patient to the attending physician; we physically examine the patient together and continue to review all data available to us which includes: laboratory values, imaging study results and notes/recommendations from other medical specialists. We use all this information to then formulate a treatment plan. This treatment plan changes throughout the day depending on the patients' clinical status.

Throughout the day I consult the intensive care team to evaluate patients within other areas of the hospital who may be showing signs of clinical deterioration and for new patients brought in by Emergency Medical Services (EMS) to the Emergency Department. My colleagues and I are part of the Rapid Response Team who attempt to prevent a deteriorating patient from having a cardiac or respiratory arrest. We also are the Code Team who attempts to resuscitate those patients in cardiac arrest.

Critically ill patients may present with multiple organ dysfunction or multi-organ failure and require mechanical ventilation for breathing assistance, vasoactive medications for blood pressure support and broad spectrum antibiotics to treat their infections. Many of our patients require central venous access. We do this by inserting an IV line into a large vein to deliver medications and to draw blood, as well as to place IV lines into arteries for accurate blood pressure monitoring. PAs insert all these lines.

Although these interventions are invasive, they often save the patient's life. It is my responsibility to assess a patient's need for these interventions, discuss them with the patient and their family, and provide them with the highest level of care. Some of our patients are elderly, and these interventions are not within their wishes. Whatever the patients decide they want for care, this is their right and we respect their decision. This allows us to formulate a different treatment plan that is suitable specifically for them to meet their needs.

My day continues with discussing any new findings with the attending physician and the critical care team and communicating this to each patient and his or her family. I also continue to interpret and order all the tests necessary to ensure our diagnosis and treatment are correct.

My day usually ends at 7:30pm. At this time, I relay the day's events, present new patients to the overnight team and go home to rest and return the next day. My schedule is six shifts every two weeks... yes eight days off, which allows for flexibility and free time to de-stress and take care of any personal responsibilities.

Career Outlook

According to U.S. News and World Report, PAs rank #1 in Best Healthcare Jobs and #3 in Best Jobs. Analysts predict a 31% employment growth in this field from 2018 to 2028, leading to 37,000 new jobs. PAs have a very low unemployment rate of around 0.8%. The 25% best paid PAs make $124,2000, while the lowest-paid 25% make $87,980.

Search and Explore

The American Academy of PAs
   https://www.aapa.org/

National Commission on Certification of Physician Assistants
   http://www.nccpa.net/

Physician Assistant Education Association
   http://paeaonline.org/

US News and World Report Best PA Programs
   https://www.usnews.com/best-graduate-schools/top-health-schools/physician-assistant-rankings

Similar Careers

Physician

Pharmacist

Nurse Practitioner

CHAPTER 9

Veterinarian

Robin K. Solomon, DVM

Education:	Bachelor's Degree	4 years
	DVM/VMD Degree	4 years
	Internship/Residency	1 - 4 years
	Fellowship/Additional	0 - 4 years
License:	North American Veterinary Licensing Examination (NAVLE))	
Median Income:	$93,830 (range, $73,000 to $162,450)	

Why I Became a Veterinarian

At a young age, I was inspired by the autobiographical stories of James Herriot, a mixed animal veterinarian in 1940s England. I was enchanted by his narratives describing how he treated all the creatures presented before him. My first job was at a local veterinary hospital where I felt a real connection with animals. Although I was only 16, I learned to approach the animals with a gentle, calm and reassuring attitude. It was a very rewarding feeling — I felt so happy when the sick cats and dogs I cared for were able to go home to their owners' loving homes. I learned that I wanted to take care of the animals as if they were my own. Pursuing an animal science major in college provided a broad knowledge base in the biology, anatomy and physiology of many animal species. During college, I milked cows at the campus dairy (and shoveled piles of manure) and gained experience with other farm animals. In my heart, I recognized a desire to care for animals. As a result of these experiences, I knew I wanted to learn all I could about all animal species, so I could be like James Herriot.

Overview

Veterinarians are the only doctors trained to protect the health and well-being of animals, and people. Veterinarians not only need to have a love for animals, but also must be able to problem-solve and have strong leadership and communication skills. The profession also demands that you stay up-to-date with the ever-expanding knowledge base. Everyday is an opportunity to learn a new skill or a better way to keep everyone healthy.

You can begin to prepare as early as middle school or high school if you think you are interested in a career in veterinary medicine. To do this, you should take as many mathematics, chemistry, biology and physics courses that are available to you. It is never too early to start preparing for the many career opportunities in college, with a sound foundation in math and science.

Specialties and Subspecialties

General Clinical Practice: This is probably what most people associate with veterinary medicine-the doctor who takes care of their pet dog, cat, guinea pig or horse. Most (about two-thirds) of veterinarians work in private practice. There are also veterinarians who focus only on food animals (such as dairy and beef cattle) or wildlife. Some veterinarians work with a combination of species. General practitioners are proficient in the basic medicine, surgery and preventative health of animals.

Specialty Clinical Practice: Some veterinarians choose to continue their education beyond the veterinary school's four-year program by completing an internship and residency program. One follows this route to become specialized or "board certified." When becoming specialized, the focus is on one area such as surgery or internal medicine of small and large animals. There are over 20 specialties in veterinary medicine. Some specialties include: cardiology, surgery, neurology, behavior and/or shelter medicine.

Research Veterinarians: These veterinarians make contributions to animal and human health by finding new ways to diagnose, treat and prevent diseases. They work in the pharmaceutical and biomedical industries, universities and in governmental agencies. Veterinarians work collaboratively with human doctors and researchers all over the world.

Public Health: Veterinarians work for city, county, state and federal agencies to investigate animal and human disease outbreaks. These veterinarians are also known as epidemiologists. They also help ensure that the food supply is safe, and work to contain and eliminate disease outbreaks.

Regulatory Medicine: Various state and government agencies employ veterinarians to prevent introducing foreign diseases into the U.S. and ensure that only healthy animals enter the food supply. Veterinarians are also involved in enforcing humane laws for treating animals in research and agriculture. The Centers for Disease Control (CDC), Environmental Protection Agency (EPA) and FDA are just a few of the organizations that rely on veterinarians to fulfill their missions.

Military Service: Various branches of the U.S. military employ veterinarians in activities such as bioterrorism surveillance, improving food safety and caring for working dogs and other animals on military bases around the world.

Veterinarians can also work for colleges, universities, professional schools, social advocacy organizations, museums, zoos, historical sites, among others.

Requirements

To be admitted into veterinary school, you must fulfill certain prerequisite class requirements which are usually achieved through a four-year undergraduate degree. Required classes normally include advanced math, basic sciences such as biology, chemistry and physics and animal science. Other factors for admission into veterinary school include experience working with animals, letters of recommendation and GRE scores. Some schools require an interview.

Presently there are 30 veterinary schools in the U.S. which confer the DVM (Doctor of Veterinary Medicine) degree. The exception is the University of Pennsylvania, which confers a VMD degree (short for the Latin term Veterinariae Medicinae Doctoris). The DVM and VMD degrees are equivalent.

All veterinary schools are four-year courses of study. Students are taught the anatomy, physiology, diseases, medicine and surgery of companion animals (e.g., cats, dogs), food animals, and exotic and wildlife species. Additionally, students learn how animal and human health are linked. During veterinary school, students split their time between class work, exams and 'hands-on' time with all animal species. Students achieve the 'hands-on' time through opportunities available early in the veterinary education process and through clinical rotations and externships in the later years of veterinary school.

All veterinarians must pass the North American Veterinary Licensing Examination (NAVLE) and fulfill the licensing requirements for the state in which they want to work. Full licensure allows you to practice as a veterinarian.

You may obtain other certification if you choose to specialize in a certain area of veterinary medicine. To become "board certified" or specialized, you must complete a one year internship. Veterinary schools or specialty veterinary hospitals offer these internships. These programs allow further training, exposure and experience in advanced veterinary care. The next level of elective training for board certification is a three-year residency, where the focus is specifically on your area of interest (either at a veterinary school or specialty practice). The final step is passing the board examination (a comprehensive evaluation of one's expertise) in that chosen specialty. Once you fulfill the required credentials, you become a diplomat (member) of that specialty group ("college").

To remain a veterinarian requires that you stay up-to-date with the ever-expanding knowledge base. All states require formal CE through conferences, webinars or other sources. However, every day is an opportunity to keep growing as a professional- to learn a new skill or be exposed to new diagnostic tests and treatments.

A Day in The Life of a Veterinarian

My day begins by attending to the hospitalized patients, evaluating treatment plans and updating owners on their pets progress. Next, I prepare for surgery by examining the pets having procedures and establishing which anesthesia I should use for each animal. I choose the appropriate medications and carefully calculate the doses for each patient. Over the next few hours, I perform cat and dog sterilization surgeries, remove a benign skin growth on a geriatric dog and extract some diseased teeth from a cat's mouth. While the animals are recovering from anesthesia, I document the procedures in their medical records, prescribe medications (such as antibiotics and pain control), and write discharge notes about home care, which I give to their owners. After a quick break for lunch, I see some scheduled appointments, including an adorable kitten adopted from a rescue group and a puppy who needs vaccine boosters to build his immunity against dangerous infectious diseases. My last appointment is one of my favorite patients, a 14-year-old cat I have taken care of since she was an 8 week old kitten. She needs some blood tests to monitor her kidney function and her thyroid function (which often change and can deteriorate as cats get older). Finally, I sit at my desk to review some test results received from the lab. After checking some textbooks and online sources, I develop management plans for these pet cases. I spend the next hour on the phone, touching base with these owners and returning the calls of some other clients who left messages for me. Once I am satisfied I have addressed the needs of the four-legged creatures and their two-legged caretakers, I can head home.

Career Outlook

Veterinarians rank #23 in Best Health Care Jobs, and #64 in the Best 100 jobs. There has been a rapid growth of veterinary jobs, with an estimated increase of about 18% through 2028. This is most likely because many more Americans are getting pets and are willing to invest in the best preventative care and state of the art diagnostics and therapies for their pets. The median veterinarian salary is around $93,830, with 15,600 new jobs and an unemployment rate of about 1.7%.

Search and Explore

American Veterinary Medical Association
http://www.avma.org

American College of Veterinary Internal Medicine
http://www.acvim.org

Humane Society Veterinary Medical Association
http://www.hsvma.org/

Veterinary Organizations and Associations
http://www.vspn.org/library/wwwdirectory/organizations.htm

Similar Careers

Agricultural and Food Scientists - Bachelor's degree

Animal Care and Service Workers - High school diploma or equivalent

Medical Scientist - Doctoral or Professional degree

Physician - Doctoral or Professional degree

Veterinary Assistants and Laboratory Animal Caretakers -

   High school diploma or equivalent

Veterinary Technologist and Technicians - Associate's degree

Zoologists and Wildlife Biologists - Bachelor's degree

CHAPTER 10

Phlebotomist

J. Spencer Verner, RN

Education:	Community College, Technical School OR on the job	4-8 months
Certification:	American Medical Technologists (AMT) or the National Center for Competency Testing (NCCT)*	
Median Income:	$34,480 (Range $25,020 - $49,060)	

Not all phlebotomy jobs require certification, wage varies based on experience, geographical location and other factors.

Why I Became a Phlebotomist

I first learned to draw blood when I was 18 years old as a Hospital Corpsman in the U.S. Navy. At that time, learning the skill was a key part of my training as a corpsman in my Navy career. After I was discharged from the Navy, I continued to work as a phlebotomist at the American Red Cross and in various hospitals and clinics.

The phlebotomist profession is not a glorious position but a skillful and professional one. You are a highly valued member of the medical team who patients often remember. In learning phlebotomy skills, I learned not only the various tricks and techniques that made me a much sought out member of the team, but one who various patients looked forward to seeing. Getting stuck in the arm with a needle is not an enjoyable experience for anyone; however, developing trust in your phlebotomy technician is valuable and knowing that the phlebotomist will make the experience less painful and frightening for the patient, is one of the greatest things I have learned over the years.

Overview

Phlebotomists, also known as phlebotomy technicians, work in a variety of settings that include not only hospitals, but also medical clinics, clinical laboratories and the American Red Cross. Patients and individuals who require blood drawing (phlebotomy) include severely ill patients to people who come into the doctor's office for yearly physicals, pre-employment screening, employees screened for work-place exposures to dangerous substances, service members screened for deployment overseas, employees and others who require an evaluation for illicit drug/toxicology use, for therapeutic drug (medication) monitoring and blood donors.

Phlebotomists are responsible medical professionals and must adhere to the same code of professional conduct as their peers. This includes refraining from illicit substance abuse, maintaining patient confidentiality and always behaving in a discreet, professional and sensitive manner when completing their task. Phlebotomists are exposed to blood and sharp objects that can injure a person if they are mishandled. Keeping up to date in handling blood and sharp medical equipment and what to do if an accident occurs is crucially important.

Responsibilities

There are not any specialties or subspecialties within the phlebotomy profession, but phlebotomists can develop their skill to a high degree. This includes improving their ability to obtain blood from patients whose veins are hard to find or obtain blood from pediatric patients who require phlebotomists to be especially skilled and compassionate. In high volume environments where there are large numbers of patients, the phlebotomist must not only be keenly skillful, but have the ability to maintain his or her composure and poise.

Requirements

Phlebotomists can obtain training in a variety of community colleges and technical schools throughout the country. It is important to receive training in a facility that is accredited by organizations, like the National Accrediting Agency for Clinical Laboratory Sciences (NAACLS), which ensures that the program is suitable to train you with all the current concerns and information you need to know about phlebotomy. Less common but also acceptable in many cases is on the job training at hospitals, the armed forces, clinics and for-profit institutions.

Phlebotomists are not licensed but any of the following agencies certify them: American Certification Agency (ACA), American Medical Technologists (AMT), American Society for Clinical Pathology (ASCP), National Center for Competency Testing/Multi-skilled Medical Certification Institute (NCCT/MMCI), National Credentialing Agency (NCA) and the National Health Career Association (NHA). However, at present, all but four states do not require phlebotomists to be certified. Yet, although phlebotomists are not required to be certified to practice, many employers may require their phlebotomists to be certified by one of the above mentioned agencies.

A Day in the Life of a Phlebotomist

Sometimes the day starts early, usually at the crack of dawn, but sometimes in the middle of the night. Phlebotomists work around the clock. I start the shift checking all the supplies in the tray that contains the equipment I will need. These include, but are not limited to syringes, blood bottles, finger lancets, gauze, band aids, alcohol preps, tourniquets and needles. The good phlebotomist is a prepared one and is ready for anything. I check the patient roster for the day. There is a terminally ill man I know on the list. Last night he came close to dying. Also, there are a few children on the hospital's pediatric wing on the list. I know it is going to be busy and I make sure that I have enough supplies to get through my rounds without having to resupply in the middle of the day.

When I enter the ward where the terminally ill man is, some of the nurses and doctors who know me wave to me. They are relieved that I have arrived. Many of them do not know how to draw a blood specimen from their patients and have been waiting some time for me to arrive. On the roster at the main nursing station desk there are a few more patients' names. I will be here a bit longer than I thought. That's okay. It is part of the job...

As I enter the patient's room, I ensure that I am projecting the sort of image I would want to see if *I* were the patient. I smile and introduce myself. The patient's wife smiles but the patient looks worried. I tell him a little about my experience and let him sort things out. To be a successful phlebotomist requires strong people skills. Allowing patients and their families to process their reservations about what is about to occur is a big part of the job.

After I am finished, I can see the patient calming down. The needle stick didn't hurt much, and I have not compromised the patient's dignity. I've done my job well and he will look forward to seeing me in the future. A nurse offers me a donut on the way out of the ward.

In the pediatric area, the three-year-old I am about to see is in his room with his dad. When he sees me, he begins to pout. I speak softly and tell the patient about what I intend to do. I move slowly and carefully as I put the tourniquet on the little arm and feel for a vein. The young patient is apprehensive: he has been hurt in the past and is antsy. I make a joke and smile reassuringly. His dad gets involved, holding the young boy in his lap as I proceed. I put the needle into the arm and a small splash of blood appears in the tubing that will take the blood from his arm to the bottle. This is a good sign. I pull the needle out a fraction, perhaps a millimeter, and the blood starts to slowly fill the bottle. Suddenly, the child jumps and the needle comes out of the arm. No worries here. I snap the needle shut and give a wad of absorbent gauze to the dad. I look at the bottle. It is half full—not ideal, but plenty to perform the needed test. I know this from experience. No loss here. Soon the child is clean and happy, and I have regained my composure. I need to...there are two more children left to see.

By the end of the day I have seen 53 patients, quite a busy day. Most of the patients were easy sticks, meaning that I was able to draw blood from them without much complication. There were four difficult cases where I was unsuccessful. All in all, a busy and successful day.

When I return home, I can relax and be content, knowing that I did my job well. I kept my cool and did as good a job as I could. Tomorrow it will be much the same as today, full of ups and downs, tests of my patience and my expertise and my ability to complete my tasks in a timely fashion.

The job is tough sometimes but that's alright. I am a professional, you know.

Career Outlook

According to U.S. News and World Report, Phlebotomists Rank #15 in Best Health Care Support Jobs and #91 in 100 Best Jobs. They report a median salary of $34,480, with a 3.3% unemployment rate. The Bureau of Labor Statistics projects a 23% employment growth for phlebotomists between 2018 and 2028, with an estimate of 29,500 new jobs.

Search and Explore

The American Society of Phlebotomy Technicians
  https://www.aspt.org/

The National Phlebotomy Association
  http://nationalphlebotomy.org/

National Association of Phlebotomists
  http://www.phlebotomy.org/

Similar Careers

Nurse

Nurses Aid

Dental Assistant

Medical and Clinical Lab Technologist and Technicians

Medical Assistant

Medical Records and Health Information Technician

Veterinary Assistant or Technician

CHAPTER 11

Dentist

Paul Albicocco, DMD, MS

Education:	Bachelor's Degree	4 years
	DMD/DDS Degree	4 years
	Internship/Residency	1-2 years
	Fellowship (optional)	0-6 years
Certification/license:	Dentistry License	
Median Income:	$156,240 (range, $72,840 - $208,000)	

Why I Became a Dentist

For me, the inspiration to become a dentist started at a very young age. The thought that someday I would be in the health field providing care in the very same practice that I visited as a child would be a dream come true. As a child who loved candy, I spent a great deal of time in the dental chair. Almost every visit, I would watch my dentist taking care of me and could tell he was having fun. It even looked as if he enjoyed what he was doing! When I became older,

I volunteered to help out at my dentist's office. I admired all the instruments and gadgets that he had for treating patients. The one thing that I noticed very early on was that the dentist needed to problem solve and provide treatment for many different situations. Throughout my years as a young adult, I was very creative and artistic. I loved building model airplanes and cars. I watched my older brother go to medical school, then work in a hospital. I would wonder if I could enter a field where I could have my own office and use my creative skills to provide medical treatment to patients outside the hospital setting. My goal was to identify a medical field where I could have my own private practice, schedule my own hours, while having the financial ability to provide for my family. I was often told that dentistry would provide a great living, and it would utilize my problem-solving skills and artistic abilities, along with medical knowledge, which would enable me to become a great dentist. Growing up in a New York City suburb, I always looked to make a living serving my community in the field of medicine. While I was in college taking tests and fulfilling the requirements for admission into dental school, I would ask myself a simple question, "Am I good enough to get accepted, and do I have what it takes to be a dentist?" I would always remember to simply look around at everyone else who was applying and remember, "You may not be better than anyone else, but no one is better than you." If your dream is to become a dentist, then go for it.

Most people think that dentists just remove teeth, fill cavities and relieve pain associated with infected teeth, but a dentist is so much more. The field of dentistry is always introducing new scientific breakthroughs that preserve patient's smiles and their self-esteem. Not only is a dentist's role to address teeth/mouth injuries and malformations, but also to diagnose and treat head and neck diseases. A dentist may also perform surgical tooth extractions and insert crowns and dental implants. Dentists also use care and attention to detail in restoring patient's dentition using the very latest, up-to-date methods. A new technique of three-dimensional-type printing uses ceramics to design and manufacture crowns, making tooth replacement possible. Over the past few years technology truly has changed dental practice. Computers have digitalized many aspects of the profession. Digital radiographs (x-rays), electronic patient charting and high tech scanners that design crowns and veneers, are some popular uses of dentistry digitalization. High quality external crown and filling manufacturing now can offer patients the highest standards of care. Some dentists do not have an interest in designing crowns or fillings. For these practitioners, they have the option to send digital images to a dental laboratory where technicians make the crowns or fillings and then they deliver the final product back to the dentist and hence to the patient.

Specialties and Subspecialties

There are nine dental specialties which you can undertake after graduating from dental school, and once completed, confer completion of a residency program. These specialties include: Dental Public Health, Endodontics, Oral and Maxillofacial Pathology, Oral and Maxillofacial Radiology, Oral and Maxillofacial Surgery, Orthodontics and Dental Facial Orthopedics, Pediatric Dentistry, Periodontics and Prosthodontics.

Dental Public Health: includes the science of preventing and controlling diseases associated with the mouth through organized community efforts. Their goal is also to promote public dental health awareness and education using applied dental research;

Endodontics: includes the health and treatment of the dental pulp which is the center of the tooth comprised of living tissue and cells. Endodontics focuses on studying normal dental pulp, and disease and injury to this tissue;

Oral and Maxillofacial Pathology: is associated with identifying and managing the mouth and the maxillofacial region (e.g., the jaw, face), with an emphasis on investigating the causes, processes and effects of these diseases. Clinical radiology, microscopy, and biochemical principles are also applied;

Oral and Maxillofacial Radiology: is associated with interpreting radiological (e.g., X-Ray) images used in diagnosing and managing oral and maxillofacial diseases;

Oral and Maxillofacial Surgery: is associated with the diagnosis and surgical treatment of diseases, defects and injuries that involve both function and beauty concerns of both hard and soft tissue (e.g., palate);

Orthodontics and Dentofacial Orthopedics: is associated with diagnosing and correcting misaligned teeth, and dealing with neuromuscular and skeletal abnormalities (See Orthodontist Chapter);

Pediatric Dentistry: is associated with comprehensive dental care for infants, children and adolescents;

Periodontics: is associated with the preventing, diagnosing and treating the supporting and surrounding tissues of the teeth, including the gums;

Prosthodontics: is associated with designing, manufacturing, and fitting artificial teeth and other parts of the mouth;

There are also fellowships and additional training in specialty areas which you can complete after graduating from dental school. There are many different specialties, each one with its own requirements that you need to fulfill in order to become a "Fellow." Most of these programs include research and teaching components.

Requirements

If you are in high school and want to become a dentist, the American Dental Education Association (ADEA) has posted an hour long webinar on how to prepare for a career in dentistry which you can access using the link: https://www.youtube.com/watch?v=bXMAQzViq-8. Once in college, most dental schools do not require students to major in the health sciences; however, it is recommended that you attend college and take classes in general biology, general and organic chemistry. After completing these prerequisite classes, the ADEA recommends applying for and taking the dental admissions test (DAT). The DAT tests Natural Sciences (Biology, General Chemistry and Organic Chemistry), Reading Comprehension, Quantitative Reasoning and administers the Perceptual Ability Test. ADEA recommends dental school applicants take the DAT at least one year before they want to go to dental school (most dental school applicants take the DAT after their junior year of college). While going through the dental school application process, you should interview with your local dental school administrator to put a face to the person on the application. This meeting can occur while in college, but preferably before your senior year, to ensure you have met all the requirements for dental school application. At the time of this writing, there were 66 dental schools in the U.S. (plus 10 in Canada) that are all current ADEA members, providing both public (e.g., state) and private education.

Following successful completion of four years of dental school, you must successfully pass the national board examination for licensure. Some states require graduating students to complete a one-year residency program at a hospital prior to obtaining their license. At this point, a new dentist can practice as a general dentist or go into a specialty program. Dentists work in many settings including public health agencies, hospitals and the military. As a General Dentist you are trained in all the specialties of dentistry and on any given day you are treating any number of oral conditions. The American Dental Association (ADA) is the nationwide organization that is the voice of dentists and a liaison to the public.

Overview

There are many reasons to choose dentistry as a career. Dentistry has been ranked as one of the most respected fields in medicine for many years and has been one of the top ten best overall professions ranked nationally in the U.S. According to the U.S. News and World Report 100 Best Jobs of 2019, Dentistry is rated #4. Dentistry is ranked #2 in Best Healthcare Jobs. Dentistry offers an opportunity to make a difference in your patients' health and well-being. It is a career that allows you to be your own boss or be part of a larger practice where you are not the boss, so you do not need to worry about the duties of running a private practice. The Bureau of Labor Statistics predicts employment growth of 7% between 2018 and 2028, with 11,600 new openings. According to this report, the median salary for a dentist was $156,240 in 2018. The best-paid 25% of dentists made $208,000, and the lowest-paid 25% made $104,800.

A Day in The Life of a Dentist

My day begins by reviewing patient charts for today's appointments and meeting with my staff to go over the schedule. I also address any emergencies that may have occurred while the office was closed. In General Dentistry, I am trained in all the specialties of dentistry, but if I am not comfortable treating a particular patient, I can always refer him or her to a specialist, so they receive the highest standard of care. I usually schedule most surgeries, such as difficult tooth extractions or implant placements, early in the morning. I could have Mrs. Jones in one room with a wisdom tooth extraction, and in another room, I could have Mrs. Smith having an x-ray to see why a tooth is hurting. Mrs. Jones's extraction went well and now it's off to check on Mrs. Smith's x-ray to see what is causing the pain. The x-ray shows an infection in the tooth nerve. Since the goal is to save the tooth, we start a root canal making the patient comfortable and pain free. In another room, the hygienist is cleaning another patient's teeth and giving her instructions on how to keep her smile beautiful and healthy. After the hygienist does the cleaning, I enter the exam room to check if the patient has any cavities and if her soft tissue is healthy. I also ensure that the patient does not have oral cancer. While all this is happening, the staff seats the next patient who I was told broke a front tooth and is very upset because she has a dinner date later this evening. I evaluate the broken tooth and decide that the tooth requires a crown so the patient can smile again and feel better. I prepare the tooth and scan the image into the computer, which designs a porcelain crown. I then send the specs to the mill, which makes the crown. While the crown is milling in the 3-D printer, I have just enough time to take some teeth impressions for a patient who needs his teeth straightened with clear braces or aligners. Once the crown is completed, I insert it onto the tooth and the patient is happy with her new restored smile. I then re-assure her that she can now enjoy her date without lacking self-confidence. Wow! It's been a busy morning. After lunch, I have Mr. Adams coming in for his dental bridge which will restore missing teeth on the upper left side of his mouth. After I place the crowns, I make him an oral appliance, like a mouth guard or retainer, to help him sleep and prevent snoring. It may be more for his wife than for him, but either way, it will make them both happy. After more patients have cleanings with the hygienist, and I perform oral examinations, it's time to provide care to patients needing a few white fillings. White fillings are tooth-colored mixtures that restore decayed teeth after I remove the decay. It is getting late and it is almost time to leave. Before we leave for the day, we call all the patients from the morning who had surgeries to ensure that they are comfortable and we ask them if they have any questions or concerns. We check to ensure that we have received the laboratory deliveries (e.g., veneers, implant crowns, dentures) that we need for the next day, and that they are ready for their respective patients. It's been a busy and fulfilling day and I can't wait to see what tomorrow brings.

I always tell patients that to me dentistry is like a hobby with which I can make a living. If you are excited about your job/career when you go to work, and it never really feels like work, then you have made the right career choice. Part of your career goal should always include giving back to the community. In my practice, I have used my skills in assisting law enforcement in identifying missing persons and identifying missing persons during the recovery efforts of September 11, 2001. As a general dentist, we use the dentition of the recovered remains and compare them to the x-rays, fillings and any other patient records when the victim was still alive. The comparison of the patients' records helps to determine their identity. As a volunteer Forensic Dentist, the work I participated in has always been very interesting, and I know that I helped many families through the healing process. To me, there is nothing more rewarding than making a positive difference in someone's life. As a dentist, I know that I have made a difference.

Career Outlook

A comfortable salary, a good work-life balance and a low unemployment rate of 0.9%, make dentistry a top career.

Search and Explore

The American Dental Association
http://www.ada.org

The American Dental Association Student membership
https://www.ada.org/en/member-center/join-or-renew-ada-membership/dental-student-membership

The National Dental Association
http://www.ndaonline.org/

American Dental Education Association
http://www.adea.org/

The American Student Dental Association
https://www.asdanet.org/

Similar Careers

Dental Hygienist

CHAPTER 12

Dental Hygienist

Catherine Monchik, RDH, BA

Education:	Associate Degree	2-3.5 years
	OR	
	Bachelor's Degree (Applied Science in Dental Hygiene)	4 years
License:	The Commission on Dental Competency Assessments (CDCA) - ADEX Dental Hygiene examination	
Median income:	$74,820 (range: $51,930 to $101,820)*	

*Some practices offer compensation on the percentage of production you create for the day instead of a salary. There can be perks such as vacation time, sick pay, medical benefits and/or incentive bonuses all to promote the employee to work to their fullest ability.

Why I Became a Dental Hygienist

My experience at the dentist was always pleasant and I had a female dentist who was a great influence on my decision to become a dental hygienist. As a young child, my dentist was one of the first women I would see working and running her own business. This was uncommon in my family as most women stayed at home. I was captivated by the hygienist and that motivated me to go into the field of dentistry. *I knew what I wanted to do at the age of two and a half!* I was her patient, and when I received my working papers (at age 15), she became my mentor, as I became her employee. While working in this field as a dental assistant, I realized how nervous patients are when they are at the dentist, and I always loved the challenge of making them feel comfortable. I find my true joy in treating children, especially those with disabilities. These children seem to need the most hygiene care which requires considerable patience.

I worked as a dental assistant before entering New York City College of Technology to pursue formal training as a dental hygienist. After I received my Associate's Degree and started my career as a hygienist, I also continued my education and earned my Bachelor's Degree in Health Administration. This degree enabled me to teach as an adjunct Clinical Professor at the college while still working as a dental hygienist. There are so many opportunities in the field of dentistry—the more education you have, the more doors open.

My advice to anyone choosing this career path is to treat each patient individually and with respect and gentleness. This is how I keep it fresh and exciting. Each patient is different. Some patients will have perfectly beautiful teeth and others may be very self-conscious and embarrassed about their teeth. I've always had compassion, and I try to make my patients feel comfortable. I can't believe 13 years later, I can say I still love being a dental hygienist and it never feels like it's a job! Also, keep learning—you will be amazed at how fast things change and improve.

Overview

A dental hygienist is a professional who performs dental services to maintain mouth health. This includes reviewing the patient's medical history, performing dental prophylaxis (preventative care) by carefully removing plaque which is soft biofilm (a bacterial mass) that builds on the teeth's surface. If this film is not removed by flossing and brushing, it will harden over time and become calculus which is a calcified deposit. During this prophylaxis, we remove plaque, calculus and stains. We perform an examination of the head and neck which would include finding any abnormalities inside the mouth, as well as examining the head and neck for any abnormalities. Dental hygienists can also take radiographs (X-ray films) on a patient and prepare the images for the dentist. These radiographs are now digital with instantaneous results. However, only the dentist can read the radiographs and diagnose the patient from the results. Dental hygienists also take teeth impressions and apply sealants. This mostly takes place on children with newly erupted permanent molars. The profession uses sealants to seal the pits or grooves on the teeth surface, to protect them from cavities and decay.

A dental hygienist can practice in a dental office setting, which is traditional, but also in a hospital, an equipped school or public institution under the general supervision of a licensed dentist. Graduates can practice dental hygiene in the armed services, in dental schools or even working for dental companies selling products such as dental supplies, preventive care products, and dental instruments.

Specialities and Subspecialities

Office setting: This type of practice is a more traditional setting of a private or insurance practice. Staff may include one or two dentists, an office manager, a few assistants and a few hygienists.

Hospital setting: This is usually a dental clinic that accepts insurance and sliding scale payments from patients who cannot afford dental treatment. This practice would have a much larger staff, including many dentists, assistants, hygienists, front office staff and administrative personnel.

Equipped school setting: A dental hygienist would be teaching in a dental hygiene college-based clinic. This setting would include a class of dental hygiene students with other clinical professors with the appropriate credentials (e.g., a bachelor's degree to teach in the clinic; a master's degree to teach lectures). A dentist must be present in each clinic.

Mobile dentistry setting: This would be a dental office "on the go." It would be in a mobile unit, such as in a recreational vehicle, or trailer and could go anywhere to give access and provide care to people in need. Mobile dentistry units can be in a school gym or other large spaces, the location can change from day to day.

Dental Sales Representatives: This practice would be working for a manufacturer selling dental products. The person in this role could be a dental hygienist with a bachelor's degree in any field with a dental hygiene license. Usually this is a full-time salaried job, with benefits. The representative would go to different dental practices introducing new dental products with the goal of selling these new products to dental practices/offices.

Requirements

To obtain a license to practice in the state of New York (where I work), you must graduate from an accredited dental hygiene program. You will need to pass state regulated exams administered by the CDCA and ADEX, with no less than a 75% grade. The grades and examinations vary from state to state. Once you are licensed in one state, you may need to retake some of the boards if you should choose to practice in a different state.

Licensing a dental hygienist in local anesthesia and nitrous oxide is now available in some states with guidelines for each state.

The degree necessary to work as a dental hygienist is an associate's degree in Applied Science in Dental Hygiene. One can also obtain a bachelor's degree, or a bachelor's degree plus a master's degree in Dental Hygiene. These credentials give the individual the ability to teach dental hygiene courses in a college.

Other degrees that one can obtain after an associate's degree in dental hygiene include: Public Health, Health Administration and Business. These fields create more opportunities for the hygienist to work. Some of these other opportunities include dental clinics or a non-profit organization providing services for the underprivileged community, dental administration or dental sales. Some hygienists might also participate in forums and group meetings to test new products.

To maintain your license, you are required to participate in mandatory CE courses. You can complete some on-line, but you must obtain the majority on-site through conferences and other sources. The law mandates that an infection control prevention course be completed every four years, and one must renew Cardiopulmonary Resuscitation (CPR) certification every two years. In the lifetime of the dental hygiene career, one child abuse prevention course must be taken.

A Day in the Life of a Dental Hygienist

The primary and traditional place for a hygienist to practice is in a clinical office setting. I arrive early to review my patients' charts and determine their plan of care for the day, whether it be radiographs, fluoride treatments, applying sealants, and/or other medical updates. The night before, I stock-up and sterilize my operatory or assigned room where I will work the following day, so I am ready when I arrive early in the morning. When a patient arrives, I go to the front of the office, take his or her chart and walk him or her to my room. I give the patient a few minutes to settle in by talking about what's new and then invite them to have a seat. I review the medical history and ask if he or she is having any dental pain since their last visit. It is important to establish a good rapport with my patient to make them feel comfortable. If my patient is experiencing any pain, I will take any necessary radiographs. I perform different treatments including dental prophylaxis (prevention). I also review dental home management with the patient, which is the most important. Subsequently, I update the patient's medical history and ask if there are any other issues to discuss. I record everything in the patient's chart and in the electronic computer record in our dental practice. The dentist then enters the exam room to perform the oral exam. He examines inside the mouth for any tooth decay or abnormalities, and performs an exam outside the mouth. In doing this exam, he looks at the head and neck region for any lesions (e.g., cancerous) or other abnormalities. After the exam is complete, I ensure that I have scheduled another appointment with this patient, which is usually six months from the current appointment (if the patient is in good health). If there are any issues, I schedule a follow-up appointment for three months. After the patient leaves, I disinfect the room, sterilize the instruments, and prepare the room for the next patient.

Once a week, I work as a clinical adjunct professor at the New York City College of Technology, where I have the pleasure of teaching future dental hygiene students. I arrive early to the clinic. Before clinic, students are sterilizing and setting up their cubicles. Clinical activities can consist of students performing dental hygiene on each other's mouths, doing paperwork, learning dental instrumentation, learning procedures and treating (non-student) patients. The students begin by taking blood pressure measurements and reviewing a patient's medical history. The students document these parameters in both a paper and electronic chart. I come in and review the medical history with the patient to ensure everything is correct and sign-off to the student. The student then does a detailed and complete patient work-up. The student performs all dental charting related to their patients' exams, and informs patients of their home dental hygiene care routine. I then review each student's paperwork for accuracy and decide a course of treatment for the patient, which the student will convey to the patient. The student then gives the treatment(s). I assess the students' work for each patient after the treatment is completed. A discussion takes place with the student regarding the exam findings, for example, if calculus is not removed or if the student did well to move on to further treatments with that patient. These discussions take place out of earshot from the patient, where they are not present. I ask if the student needs assistances, and if they do, I help. Sometimes "show-tell-do" works in helping the student select and use the correct instrument. I collect their folders and the students sterilize their used equipment.

Career Outlook

According to the Bureau of Labor Statistics, Dental Hygienists rank #2 in Best Health Care Support Jobs and #30 in their 100 Best Jobs ranking. They estimate that the dental hygiene occupation will grow 11% by 2028, with an estimated 23,700 new jobs. This is faster than the average growth rate for most professions, with a very low unemployment rate of 0.4%. The increase in Dental Hygienist jobs is likely due to an increased awareness among consumers of how oral health is linked to overall health; the best-paid 25% made $88,820, while the lowest-paid 25% made $61,230. In 2018, the median salary for dental hygienists was $74,820, with a salary range of $51,930 to approximately $101,820.

Search and Explore

The American Dental Hygiene Association
   http://www.ADHA.org

The American Dental Hygiene Association Programs
   http://www.adha.org/dental-hygiene-programs

The Commission on Dental Accreditation
   http://www.ada.org/en/coda

Similar Careers

Dental Assistant - Post secondary non degree award

Medical Assistant - Post secondary non degree award

Dentist

Orthodontist

CHAPTER 13

Dietitian Nutritionist

Carolyn DiMicco, RD, CDN

Education:	Bachelor's Degree	4 years
	Master's Degree	2 years
	Internship	6-12 months
Registration:	Commission on Dietetic Registration	
Median income:	$60,370 (range, $38,460 - $84,610)	

Why I Became a Registered Dietitian Nutritionist

Food has always intrigued me. As a toddler, I frequented this tiny hole in the wall place, snuggled into the front step. It was the kind of place you go to when you crave something satisfying like a good eggplant parmesan, pasta Primavera – or my favorite – Olive Fingers (black olives atop five fingers, ready to be plucked into the mouth). Just as often, my parents often found me hiding in the cupboard with chocolate smeared across my face and cookie crumbs piled in my lap. That's right, my favorite place was the refrigerator.

As I grew into an adolescent and became more physically active, I stopped indulging in pizza and doughnuts after school, and began learning how food can fuel the body. In health class, I remember learning the basics: meals should be balanced; avoid overeating; and protein builds muscles.

Initially, I learned about dietitians when my grandfather was undergoing a process by which a machine performed the responsibility of his failing kidneys: dialysis. He had a grueling several years of bland meals devoid of salt, potassium-containing fruits, and beans. The idea that food could be medicine – just as much as it could be harmful – was intriguing to me.

After entering my dietetic program in college, I began learning more about the human body and how nutrition could influence disease states. While I initially started the program believing that I would one day be the owner of a nutrition empire bringing recipe books, TV series, and gourmet (but healthful) food to the public, I began to think that my path would lead me elsewhere. During my senior year of undergraduate studies, I decided to pursue a career as a clinical dietitian and began the process of applying for internships.

Even after becoming a registered dietitian, my career path continually changes. I have pursued several avenues and explored options that I said I "never" would. In truth, the beauty of being a dietitian is the power to adapt and change to the needs of our environment and population. After exploring my career in areas such as bariatrics, critical care, advanced nutrition support and now pediatrics, I pursued a Master's in Business Administration in healthcare administration and management recognizing that my passion for food, health and medicine complement my big ideas for healthcare management. I am dedicated to population health needs. My hope is to change health and healthcare on a broader scale, starting with pediatrics.

Overview

Registered Dietitian Nutritionists (RDNs) embody a large field of study, encompassing food and culinary arts, food science and engineering, health and wellness and clinical nutrition support. RDNs can hold a variety of jobs within their careers, including becoming a dietitian within a hospital, long-term care center, school or other facility. Additionally, RDNs can work as chefs, restauranteurs, healthcare marketers, educators, consultants or food scientists –like Alton Brown who uses a combination of chemistry and culinary arts to study existing food structures, as well as to create new food sources.

In reality, RDNs have many skills and acquire vast knowledge that prepares them for numerous positions. It is my belief that dietitians are under-utilized and under-marketed within our current healthcare system, as well as in society. If you are interested in becoming a RDN, I encourage you to constantly push yourself to learn new things – both related to food and nutrition, and not. Explore areas that do not always seem interesting or important for these can be the most riveting and rewarding. RDNs are well-equipped to establish themselves in other capacities, such as in administration, education, legislation, or program and project management.

Although there are many professions for which you can qualify with a nutrition interest or background, the medical profession, both nationally and internationally, widely respects RDNs. The Academy of Nutrition and Dietetics, a national professional organization representing and supporting credentialed nutrition practitioners, requires that RDNs are registered by The Commission on Dietetic Registration. This provides credibility to the holder in all areas of practice.

Specialties and Subspecialties

Nutrition has many fields of study. Possible specialties that require board certification to pursue are:

General Clinical Practice: As a practicing RDN, you will have the opportunity to work as a dietitian in a community setting, such as a private practice, government-funded outreach program such as Women, Infants and Children (WIC), or as part of a healthcare system. If you are working in general practice, you may work in a hospital or long-term care center as a clinical dietitian. If working for an office or private practice, you may provide counseling to clients with a range of health-related needs from normal nutrition to disease-specific medical nutrition therapy, including weight management.

Diabetic Nutrition: As you might imagine would happen with the rise of obesity in America, there is a need for Certified Diabetes Educators (CDEs). CDEs are healthcare professionals who have extensive knowledge in the management and prevention of diabetes. Expertise spans not only nutrition knowledge, but effective medicinal and other management.

Gerontological Nutrition: Gerontological nutrition is a special subtype of nutrition that specifically addresses the nutrition needs of the geriatric population. Nutrition requirements of the aged become challenging, including managing optimal nutrition and hydration in dementia, post-stroke and overall frailty. As the human body ages, it is natural to begin to lose thirst and hunger cues. Therefore, a large portion of gerontological nutrition is having competency in ethical issues surrounding feeding and hydrating elderly patients, particularly near the end-of-life.

Pediatric Nutrition: On the opposite spectrum from geriatrics is pediatrics. Just as important as it is to have a comprehensive understanding for the elderly population, it is equally important to have competency when providing care to neonates, infants and children. Contrary to popular belief, children and adolescents are not little versions of fully-grown adults. They have unique nutrition requirements for development. Perhaps the most daunting area of expertise within the world of pediatric nutrition is nutrition for neonates and infants. Children who are admitted to the neonatal and pediatric intensive care units (NICU and PICU) often require intensive nutrition therapy.

Renal Nutrition: This area of nutrition encompasses diet planning and nutrition intervention for those who are pre-dialysis or currently undergoing dialysis. Renal nutrition is complicated. However, proper nutrition is essential to successfully manage renal disease.

Oncology Nutrition: Understanding oncology nutrition is a necessity to facilitating healing and support for those either undergoing cancer treatment or who are receiving palliative care. In this area of nutrition, practitioners tend to exercise creativity when finding solutions to complex issues surrounding pain, lack of appetite, painful or difficult swallowing, altered taste, and weight loss.

Sports Dietetics: If you are thinking about providing diet advice to athletes of any age – up to the Olympic level – you should consider a career in sports nutrition. In this field of study, RDNs specialize in understanding how food can fuel the body for optimal athletic achievement.

Obesity and Weight Management: As obesity continues to plague America, weight management and bariatric nutrition are of utmost importance. The area of bariatric nutrition encompasses conventional weight management by integrating healthful eating habits, as well as specialized nutrition therapy for pre- and post-bariatric surgery (i.e. lap band surgery, sleeve gastrectomy and gastric bypass).

Nutrition Support: Nutrition support is an area of expertise that encompasses artificial nutrition, whether it is enteral or parenteral nutrition. Enteral nutrition involves artificial feeding tubes either placed into the stomach or another area of the intestine to deliver nutrients in the form of liquid formula. Parenteral nutrition tends to be a more short-term solution to artificial nutrition support, although it can be long-term as well. This type of nutrition support is delivered by IV infusion with a specialized solution containing protein, fat, glucose, electrolytes and vitamins. Each prescription is individualized for the patient. Specialized nutrition support can occur in many settings, but it is more common in the critical care setting of a hospital.

Other options for career paths that do not require board certification include: legislature, public health, food science and academia.

Requirements

To become an RDN, you must start preparing in college. RDNs are required to complete a four-year undergraduate degree in nutrition and/or dietetics that is accredited by the Accreditation Council for Education in Nutrition and Dietetics (ASCEND). Coursework includes psychology, biology, physiology, microbiology, chemistry, biochemistry, statistics, research, communication, education, food science and nutrition. If you already have an undergraduate degree in another field, often, you can make up the missing prerequisite courses to complete the required criteria for registration. Although a master's degree in nutrition and/or dietetics is not yet a national requirement for registration, it is often a preferred requirement for employment, especially in the clinical setting.

You should also begin getting involved in extracurricular activities as early as possible in your college career. After completing the undergraduate required courses, you are then required to complete a nationally accredited internship program. Each program – with a focus on clinical nutrition, community nutrition or food service – runs between six and twelve months. Internships are unpaid, and often require a fee or tuition for enrollment once you are accepted into the program. Acceptance to an internship program is becoming more competitive, since many more prospective dietitians are applying for internships with fewer spaces available. To prepare for an acceptance, you should begin volunteering, educating or becoming involved in another activity outside of schoolwork.

After successful completion of the internship program, you will be eligible to schedule your registration exam with the Commission on Dietetic Registration (CDR). A passing grade on the registration exam will qualify you for registration as an RDN, and you will be required to obtain CE credits to maintain certification throughout your career. Licensure is state-organized, and each state has differing requirements for registration. Some states in the U.S. do not require licensure to work and operate as an RDN; however, all states within the U.S. require registration through the CDR.

Once you have passed the registration exam and begin working in your field of study, you can obtain further specialty certifications. Studying required materials and coursework are a necessity to passing examinations for board certifications in specialties like nutrition support, pediatrics, and sports nutrition, to name a few.

A Day in The Life of a Registered Dietitian Nutritionist

Nowadays, my day starts off a little differently than in my recent past. I work with children who are medically complex and somewhat fragile with many diseases and medical problems (e.g. co-morbidities) who also reside in a long-term care facility. While every child at the center receives palliative care, not all the children are expected to come to the facility for end-of-life care. Palliative care simply means providing services – both conventional and not – that will foster comfort and quality of life. Many of the children who live at the center will live long lives, often outgrowing the facility's pediatric age requirement. Although there are some dark days, most of my days are filled with bright smiles and cheery dispositions shared equally by the residents and the staff members.

Every morning when I come in, I start by greeting my coworkers on the way to my desk, which is located outside of a four-bedded resident room shared by four sweet boys. After saying good morning to the children who live in the hall where my desk space is located, I begin my day by checking the current and changed diet orders for each child who resides in my neighborhood. You see, we call the units "neighborhoods" instead of "units" or "wards," hoping to foster a feeling of home. In fact, all that I do in my current position is attempt to provide a loving, warm relationship for the children in a home-like environment, within the scope of nutrition. Although this job is far from what I had originally planned I would ever do, I find it just as rewarding – if not more so – than working as a nutrition support clinician in the surgical intensive care unit.

While most of the children in my neighborhood have gastric tubes – a means of delivering artificial nutrition to individuals who do not have full use of their mouth or esophagus – I still spend plenty of time planning and delivering nutritious meals to my kids. At the Center, we have a range of children with varying chewing and swallowing abilities who may require anything from food purees to a regular-consistency diet. When working with all children, often the biggest challenge is working around food jags and preferences to provide a balanced and healthful meal that is both appealing and keeps mealtimes fun and pleasurable. A food jag is when a child will eat only one food item, or a small group of food items, for every meal.

Throughout the day, I have multiple tasks. Medical staff evaluate and assess each child in the facility on a quarterly basis. During these assessments, I check to ensure the child is both adequately nourished, and that I am helping to facilitate their medical, social, and sometimes emotional goals with nutrition support. When I am not evaluating children, I often feed them or eat my meals with them to further foster a sense of community and family mealtime, create recipes and provide input for providing a satisfying and healthful menu for each child. There is frequently much education involved in my job, whether it is educating the parents or the staff.

Finally, I end my day the same way I started it: I make the rounds to say goodnight to the children I serve each day.

Career Outlook

U.S. News and World Report ranks the career of Dietitian and Nutritionist as #86 in the 100 Best Jobs, and #25 in Best Health Care Jobs. Analysts attribute growth in this field to both the aging population, looking to stay healthy and the increasing obese population, who seek help in diet and lifestyle changes. The Bureau of Labor Statistics expects the Dietician/Nutritionist career to increase at a rate of 11% from 2018 and 2028, leading to 8,000 new jobs, with an average salary of $60,370, and a low unemployment rate of 1.5%.

Search and Explore

The Academy of Nutrition and Dietetics
http://www.eatrightpro.org

The Academy of Nutrition and Dietetics Student Member
https://www.eatrightpro.org/membership/membership-types-and-criteria/student-member

The Commission on Dietetic Registration
https://www.cdrnet.org/

United States Department of Agriculture National Agricultural Library - Dietetic Associations
https://www.nal.usda.gov/fnic/dietetic-associations

Similar Careers

Registered Nurse

Rehabilitation Counselor

Health Educator

CHAPTER 14

Orthodontist

Robert J. Peterman DMD, MDS

Education:	Bachelor's Degree	4 years
	Dental Degree (DMD or DDS)	4 years
	Orthodontic Residency	3 years
Certification:	Dentistry License	
License:	Orthodontics License	
Median Income:	$229,380 (range, $78,370 - $232,980)	

Why I Became an Orthodontist

Looking back at pictures of myself when I was 12 years old always gives me a chuckle. Like most 12-year olds, I had teeth that were far from picture-perfect. Mine were spaced out enough that I could drink with a straw through my two front teeth. It was at that age my mother took me to my local orthodontist for an evaluation. After two years of orthodontic treatment (braces), I emerged with a smile that I am still proud of today. During high school, my experience at the orthodontist encouraged me to start "shadowing" (or following) a practicing dentist, to learn more about the profession. This started me on a life path that included college, dental school, orthodontic residency, multiple board and licensure exams and most recently buying and running my own orthodontic practice.

While in high school, I spent time shadowing a dentist in a dental practice. This solidified my goal to pursue a dentistry career and then ultimately an orthodontics career. These doctors had all the qualities that I hoped to achieve in my own professional future. They are unique in that they work with their hands to solve problems, encourage their patients to be healthy and run successful businesses. They are well respected in their field. I spent my high school years building my resume for college, spending weekends learning about the various specialties in dentistry and prepping for the SATs.

College came with a new set of academic challenges. The pre-dental requirements were identical to pre-med requirements and included chemistry, biology and physics classes. All were very challenging science courses. Admission to dental school is dependent on a high grade point average (GPA) and a high score on the Dental Admission Test (DAT). Admission is highly competitive, but most schools use a single online application through the America Association of Dental Schools Application Service (AADSAS).

Overview and Requirements

Orthodontists spend seven years in academic training after finishing college. The first four of those years are in dental school. During the first two years of dental school students learn all the complexities of the human body with classes that include human anatomy, physiology, biochemistry and dental-oriented sciences. Students learn on mannequins, drill on teeth and perform all the skills dentists need to know. The final two years of dental school involve clinical work on patients and honing skills needed to become a dentist. In many schools, students often rotate through various clinics, hospitals and other community settings, while working under a clinical instructor's direct supervision. This provides students the opportunity to work closely with other health professionals and health professions students, giving them the appreciation of a team approach to healthcare delivery.

After the four years of dental school, students may apply to any of the very competitive residency programs to continue their education. The nine recognized dental specialties include: dental public health, endodontics, orthodontics, oral surgery, pediatric dentistry, periodontics, prosthodontics, oral and maxillofacial pathology and oral and maxillofacial radiology. I continued for another three years in a specialty orthodontic residency.

During orthodontic residency, students learn all facets of the specialty. Our day included screening patients in the clinic for improper bite (known as malocclusions), taking photos, x-rays and creating plaster models of patients' teeth for study. After planning how to treat our patients, we placed braces and orthodontic wires to start moving their teeth into proper positioning. We saw patients every four to six weeks for the next one to three years depending on their specific case. Orthodontic residents also learn about facial growth and development to understand how malocclusions form and how to prevent problems from developing. After completing the residency, students can apply through the American Board of Orthodontics (ABO) to take the board examination. Like most other health professions, CE is required to remain current in the field and to maintain licensure.

A Day in the Life of an Orthodontist

Working as an orthodontist is extremely rewarding. Most of my patients are teenagers, which makes each day fun and exciting. Each day I learn about the latest fads, newest teen fashion and local sporting events. On average, orthodontic treatments last about two years. During those years orthodontists often are able to see a child transform from an awkward pre-teen to a confident adolescent proud of his or her new smile. Most importantly, orthodontists can build relationships with patients and their families.

One of the most exciting parts of orthodontics today is the integration of technology into modern practice. Over the past decade, clear aligner technology, such as Invisalign®, has created an entirely new treatment process for straightening teeth. Aligners are removable, plastic trays that can move teeth without braces. Clear aligner technology has evolved to efficiently and comfortably correct many orthodontic problems. Recently, researchers have developed three-dimensional x-ray technology known as cone beam computed tomography (CBCT). These x-rays allow the orthodontist to visualize the teeth roots, bone and other facial structures with amazing accuracy. Many orthodontic offices are replacing dental impressions with digital scanners. These are highly sensitive digital cameras that image a patient's teeth creating a three-dimensional model. We use this process for study, record keeping or making orthodontic appliances.

Beyond clinical practice, most orthodontists have an excellent lifestyle compared to other medical specialties. Overall, the orthodontic population is young and usually healthy. Very few medical conditions prevent an individual from having orthodontic treatment and true medical emergencies are very rare in the orthodontic office. Most private practice orthodontists often can create their own work schedule, choosing whether or not to work nights and weekends. Orthodontists are also high earners compared to others in medical and dental professions.

Some profession negatives include increasing competition with general dentists performing some orthodontic services, which decreases the number of patient referrals to orthodontists. Additionally, dental school and orthodontic residency tuition comes with a tremendous financial cost. It is not unusual for a new orthodontist to have hundreds of thousands of dollars in student loan debt before starting practice. Finally, orthodontic training comes with the commitment of many years of school after college and an extremely stressful and competitive process while entering an orthodontic training program.

Current Career Outlook

According to U.S. News and World Report's 100 Best Jobs and Best Paying Jobs of 2019, Orthodontists rank #5. Of the U.S. News and World Report's Best Health Care jobs, Orthodontists rank #3. The U.S. Bureau of Labor Statistics reports that this profession will grow by 19.3% from 2016 to 2026, resulting in about 1,300 new job openings. Orthodontists have a median salary of $208,000, with a 0.9% unemployment rate.

Search and Explore

American Dental Education Association
http://www.adea.org/

American Association of Orthodontists
https://www.aaoinfo.org/

American Dental Association
http://www.ada.org/

American Board of Orthodontics
https://www.americanboardortho.com/

American Student Dental Association
https://www.asdanet.org/

Similar Careers:

Endodontist

Periodontist

Prosthodontist

CHAPTER 15

Podiatrist and Podiatric Surgeon

Kamilla Danilova, DPM

Education:		
	Bachelor's Degree	4 years
	Master's Degree	4 years
	Internship	3-4 years
Certification/License:	Podiatric Surgery License	
Median income:	$129,550 (range: $52,060-$282,600)	

Why I Became a Podiatrist/Podiatric Surgeon

When I was 16, I immigrated to the U.S. from the Soviet Union. I attended high school in Brooklyn where a biology teacher played a big role in my decision to pursue a medical career. I found Physiology and Biology fascinating because they provided me with answers to complicated questions about our body, function and existence within the environment. I became one of the best students in class even though I had difficulty due to my language barrier. If I only knew now that this would become a place that I would call my home, a place that gave me so many chances and so many opportunities...then I would proudly have taken every minute of those challenges that I faced back then. At the end of the semester, I realized that this was the first of many biology classes that I would be taking. This is where my medical education started and eventually led me to one of the most versatile, productive and rewarding specialties.

By the twelfth grade, I was accepted to Hunter College - City University of New York, where I pursued a bachelor of arts in Psychology, with pre-medicine courses. Hunter College was a perfect transition for me as a shy foreign girl to become a more confident, assimilated American pre-med student. During my undergraduate coursework, I met my husband and had my first son. These first several years living in New York made me stronger as a person and stronger academically. I was ready to take on the next challenge. One night, I found myself in the emergency room accompanying my husband who had severe foot pain. At that time, I was going through the application process for dental school. That busy hospital environment and the sight of young energetic doctors providing care to my husband, made me curious about their specialty. I remember asking one of the residents about her professional journey and she said, "It's a great school! You should look into it." I couldn't agree more. I investigated the New York School of Podiatric Medicine (NYSPM) that same night, applied and was accepted within two months. Now 12 years later, following four years of academics at NYSPM, three years of surgical training and five years of private practice in Manhattan; I recall memories of that first day in the American high school that to this day still seems like the most challenging day of my life. Pursuing medicine was my calling but becoming a foot and ankle specialist was my destiny.

Overview

A podiatrist is a Doctor of Podiatric Medicine (DPM). A DPM prevents, diagnoses and treats foot and ankle disorders, injuries and diseases, as well as those related to structures of the leg. A podiatrist earns a DPM degree by attending four years of Podiatry Medical School, followed by three to four years of a hospital residency. A podiatrist is the most qualified specialist for taking care of foot and ankle conditions. This involves more specialization than physicians, due to our narrow focused specialization and extended training. Podiatrists can specialize in areas such as surgery, orthopedics or public health, to name a few. Podiatrists can also subspecialize in the areas of pediatrics, sports medicine, radiology, dermatology, geriatrics or diabetic foot care. Podiatrists can work in a private or group practice, Managed Care Organizations, Preferred Provider Organizations, hospitals and extended care facilities (e.g., nursing homes, long-term care, rehabilitation centers), the U.S. Public Health Service, branches of the military (e.g., Navy, Army, Coast Guard), the VA, municipal health departments, and health professions schools.

Specialties and Subspecialties

Primary Care in Podiatric Medicine: Provides diagnosis and treatment of conditions affecting the foot, ankle and related structures of the leg (or lower extremity).

Limb Preservation and Salvage: Provides management of patients with vascular disease or diabetes, or related conditions, who are high risk for foot and leg amputation.

Diabetic Foot Wounds and Foot Wear: Provides management of patients with diabetic foot wounds, to evaluate these patients for proper footwear to prevent further complications.

Foot and Ankle Surgery: Uses modern operating procedures to improve various foot and ankle problems.

Lower Extremity Geriatric Medicine: Treatment of lower extremity disorders in the elderly.

Podopediatrics: Prevention, diagnosis and treatment of children's foot and leg problems.

Minimally Invasive Foot and Ankle Surgery: Performs surgery using the smallest possible incisions.

Podiatric Sports Medicine: The prevention, diagnosis and treatment of lower extremity disorders in athletes.

Podiatric Orthopedics (Biomechanics): Non-surgical treatment of imperfect foot and leg structure and function using special footwear, orthotics (devices that can help maintain proper foot support by realigning the foot and distributing body weight), prosthetic devices and physical therapy.

Requirements

During the four years of (podiatric) medical education, faculty teach detailed aspects of podiatric medicine and podiatric surgery to provide a sound background.

Becoming a foot and ankle specialist takes at least 11 years after finishing high school. A bachelor of science degree in Pre-Med or a bachelor of science degree is required. In addition, you must pass the MCAT in order to apply to Podiatry Medical School. Majoring in the sciences such as Biology, Chemistry or Biochemistry is an advantage but not a mandatory requirement for Podiatry School. If you obtain an average score of 24 on the MCAT and have a GPA of 3.0, you can apply. However, letters of recommendation, medical experience and research work are all contributing factors for a strong application. Presently there are nine accredited Podiatric Schools of Medicine nationwide. The curriculum is very similar to most other medical schools, where the first two years are focused in acquiring fundamental medical knowledge (didactic education), followed by two years of clinical education and medical rotations. However, for Podiatry Medicine School, the two years of clinical education and rotations are specialized in lower extremity care.

After graduating from podiatry school, you must complete a three to four-year residency. Residency training provides a combination of surgical and medical experiences. The duration of residency varies due to the extent of surgical training. By the end of residency, each candidate must obtain a state license in podiatric medicine and surgery. A podiatrist can be Board Certified in Podiatric Medicine and Podiatric Surgery.

Most podiatrists practice in an office with other medical specialists, as solo practitioners, or as hospital employees.

A Day in the Life of a Podiatrist/Podiatric Surgeon

My typical workday begins at 8:30 am. I start seeing patients at 8:45 - 9:00 am. Patients come in with various complaints, injuries and concerns. Sometimes I receive patients who require urgent care. These are patients who do not require hospitalization but urgently need a specialist's attention. These are patients who often have moderate to severe ankle sprains that require a cast or an orthopedic immobilization device. These patients could also be those with open diabetic wounds that need sharp debridement and wound care products. These patients could also have foot fractures that require immediate attention. In addition to patients with urgent care needs, I also practice general podiatry. General podiatry includes therapeutic injections for treating painful joints and ligaments, treatment of skin conditions on the foot, removal of soft tissue lesions, foot casting for custom orthotics and diabetic foot assessments. At the end of my work day, when I finish seeing patients, I review and sign all patients' laboratory and MRI results, return phone calls and prepare patient charts for upcoming surgeries. Every Tuesday I block out some time for surgical procedures such as bunion corrections (see below), hammer toe deformities, repairing ligaments and tendons, surgical wound management for diabetic wounds and various types of foot and/or toe amputations. A bunion is a bony bump that forms on the joint at the base of the big toe which causes pain. The main sign of a bunion is the big toe pointing towards the other toes on the same foot, this may force the foot bone attached to it to stick outwards. Hammer toe deformities are foot deformities that occur due to an imbalance in the muscles, tendons or ligaments that normally hold the toe straight. The type of shoes you wear, foot structure, trauma and certain disease processes can contribute or cause these to develop. Wearing proper shoes, physical therapy or surgery can correct bunions.

Additionally, I also participate in medical rounds for hospitalized patients with podiatric issues. I do this with a team of podiatry residents in the hospital, where we discuss patient care plans.

Although my specialty is very demanding, encompassing both office practice and performing surgery, it still leaves me time to spend with my family.

Career Outlook

The Bureau of Labor Statistics ranks podiatrists #17 in Best Health Care Jobs, #22 in The Best 100 Jobs, and #14 in Best Paying Jobs with a median salary of $129,550. The Bureau of Labor Statistics estimate that the practice of podiatry will increase 6% through 2028, leading to 600 new jobs, with a 1.2% unemployment rate. They estimate that the best-paid (top 25%) podiatrists earned $190,400 and the lowest-paid 25% made $83,180. Due to the increasing aging population, the Bureau of Labor Statistics predicts that more people will experience ankle- and foot-issues.

Search and Explore

The American Association of Colleges of Podiatric Medicine
http://www.aacpm.org

The American Podiatric Medical Association
http://www.apma.org

The American Podiatric Medical Association - Students and Residents
https://www.apma.org/StudentsandResidents/content.cfm?ItemNumber=27077

Council on Podiatric Medical Education
https://www.cpme.org/

The American Association of Colleges of Podiatric Medicine Residencies
https://www.aacpm.org/residencies/

The American Board of Multiple Specialties in Podiatry
https://www.abmsp.org/get_certified.php

Similar Careers

Physical Therapist

Occupational Therapist

Physician

Surgeon

Dentist

CHAPTER 16

Biomedical Engineer

Randal Chinnock, BS

Education:	Bachelor's Degree	4 years
	Master's Degree	1-2 years
	Doctor of Philosophy (optional)	3-6 years
Median income:	$88,550 (range, $51,890 to $144,350)	

Why I became a Biomedical Engineer

Like many kids in high school, I wasn't sure what I wanted for a career. My guidance counselor asked me what I liked to do.

I said, "I build things. I like to figure out how things are made."

"What things?" he asked.

"Furniture. Go-carts. Motorcycles. TVs. Tree houses".

"You sound like an engineer!" he said.

He was right. I went to college and earned a bachelor's degree in Engineering Physics. The "Engineering" part means figuring out how to solve big problems by breaking them down into small problems. The "Physics" part was the understanding of the laws of nature that make engineering possible – or impossible! (For example, nothing can travel faster than the speed of light, so don't try to design something that does). Over the years, I did many different kinds of engineering, but what I liked best was biomedical engineering (BME). That's because it gives you the opportunity to help millions of people all over the world survive diseases and recover from injuries. Eventually, I started my own company and through the years hired many people – mostly other engineers. Together, we created products that you, your family and your friends might see in a doctor's office or hospital, like arthroscopes for fixing "blown-out knees", or LASIK machines for improving vision. It is work to be proud of – creating devices to better patients' lives.

Overview

BMEs create new medical devices. A medical device is a tool that doctors, surgeons, nurses and other medical professionals use to diagnose and treat patients. A stethoscope is a simple medical device for listening to the heart and diagnosing heart and lung problems. Medical professionals use a computed tomography (CT) scanner to diagnose bone fractures and other internal problems. Practitioners use a surgical stapler to close an incision in the body after surgery. Hospitals, clinics and physician offices are full of medical devices. However, there is always a need for a better device – something that is less expensive, easier to use or more accurate. Any guess where the best ideas for new medical devices often come from? Sometimes they come from the engineers, but often they come from the users who work with these tools every day. These healthcare professionals bring ideas for improvements (or entirely new devices) to us: the engineers. From there, it is up to us to figure out how to turn those ideas into something real.

We start out by writing down *exactly* what the device needs to do in the users hands. Then we use special engineering software programs to design mechanisms to grip or move something, optical systems to light or capture images and electronic circuits that will perform the functions we need. We build rough versions of the device, called *prototypes*, that we can put in the users' hands so that they can tell us if we are on the right track. Based on what the users tell us, we refine the design, make more realistic prototypes and go through a series of tests to see if the device works properly. Sometimes there is a *human study* that we call a clinical trial, where the patients use the new device in a very careful and controlled way to ensure that the device is safe and effective. If it is, then we apply to the FDA to approve the device. Only then do we work with a manufacturer to make thousands or millions of the devices. There is nothing in the world more rewarding than a patient telling you that something you created saved his or her life.

Specialties and Subspecialties

There are many specialties within biomedical engineering. I love the BME discipline because it draws from many other engineering disciplines, such as mechanical engineering (ME), electrical engineering (EE), chemical engineering (ChemE), optical engineering (OE) and computer science or engineering (CS or CE or CSE). Biomedical engineers typically have a *concentration* or specialization in one of those areas. That means that they take more courses in one area of study. To that they add chemistry, biology and physiology studies to understand how the human body works. Some bachelor's degree programs include year-long projects where you get to come up with an idea for a new device, build a prototype and test it. If you have an ME concentration, you might end up designing knee implants, or a stair-climbing wheelchair. With an EE or CS/CE concentration, you might develop electronic devices to analyze brain waves. With a ChemE or biology concentration you might create new materials to glue wounds back together or repair the spine. OEs develop novel ways of looking inside the body with light, such as 3D high definition vision systems for surgical robots, or ways of detecting cancer with a flash of light! Some BMEs decide to work in dentistry or on veterinary devices. You can have a career with a bachelor's degree, and you don't need to go through any certification process like some professions require. However, you can choose to obtain certification in certain *skills* that BMEs use, such as in computer-aided-design (CAD), software development tools (e.g., LabView) or program management. Many employers offer post-graduate training, to which you should always take advantage. Many biomedical engineers go on to a masters degree (MS) or even a Doctor of Philosophy (Ph.D.) in order to obtain more specialized knowledge, advance their career and earn higher salaries.

Some BME jobs are in hospitals and research institutions, where they test and maintain equipment and sometimes work on new devices. However, most BMEs work for "for-profit" medical device companies. The biggest ones include Medtronic, Johnson & Johnson, General Electric and Boston Scientific. Even companies from other fields are becoming involved in producing medical devices. Google's parent company, Alphabet, is making huge investments in surgical robots, and Ford Motor Company is developing sensors in steering wheels that can monitor your vital signs as you drive. Often, the most exciting work is at a medical device *startup*. These are sometimes founded by BMEs and it can be super stimulating to work within a small group of other smart people on a common mission. The work environment is a mix of offices, research/ development labs and dust-free manufacturing areas. If you are a creative person, the product development part of the business might be for you — especially if you like using computer programs to design things and using your hands to build prototypes. If you like producing things and figuring out how to make things better, the manufacturing side could work for you. If you like to interact with people, selling the product to users might be a fit. In any of those roles, it is likely that you will work with a variety of other engineering disciplines, so you will have the chance to learn from them.

Requirements

According to a Forbes article from 2012, Biomedical Engineering is the fastest-growing college major in the U.S. However, according to this article, "These are not majors that anyone could do. They are hard, and these programs weed people out. However, there is high demand for them and a low supply of people with the skills, so it drives up the labor market price." To prepare for this major, you should focus on science, technology, engineering and math (STEM) courses in middle school and high school. If your schools don't offer many STEM courses, then you may need to take some at a community college before applying for a 4-year degree program. In some states (Massachusetts is one), if you graduate from a 2-year community college program, you are automatically accepted into the state university system (which is excellent). Whether you focus more on the science (e.g., biology), math (e.g. calculus), engineering (e.g., robotics) or technology (e.g. computer programming), classes will depend on which BME specialty you decide to pursue. Here's a little secret: when I hire BMEs, what is even more important than the BME degree is the candidate's *curiosity factor*. What have they created? Do they ask many questions? The best engineers always want to know *why*.

A Day in the Life of a Biomedical Engineer

At my company, which I founded in 1994, we specialize in developing optics-based medical devices. Examples of products that we've developed include lasers for tattoo removal, intra-oral scanners for making models of teeth and gums ("digital impressions"), catheters for seeing inside blood vessels within the heart ("intravascular imaging") and 3D high definition video-microscopes for brain surgery. We develop these novel medical devices under contract for other companies. Those companies can be startups that don't yet have the staff to develop products themselves, or big companies that may not have our expertise. I am the company's CEO, which means I spend considerable time "running the business." This means finding new business and managing the workload. However, because we're still a small company, I also contribute to product development activities. I arrive at work every weekday around 9am. My days are usually a mix of meetings and individual work. We start the day with a "scrum" where all the employees get together in the big conference room and each person takes 30-60 seconds to update the others on their activities and to identify any issues with which they may need help. We also use this daily get-together to have fun. We joke around a little and maybe share some personal news. This helps everyone feel like we're all on the same team. Later, I'll meet with my engineers and managers to discuss how a new device's design is progressing. If someone is stuck on a problem, we'll "brainstorm" (offer ideas, build on each other's ideas) to find solutions. I may speak with a customer who tells me that the prototypes we shipped to them last month are working well, and I'll share that good news with our team. I spend considerable time at my computer, doing the usual email, but also working with Computer Aided Design (CAD) programs to design a new instrument for, for example, heart surgery. Sometimes I have lunch with other employees, but other times I'm excited about what I'm working on and eat at my desk so that I can get more done. Sometimes at lunch I take a walk around the neighborhood where the company is located. I might have an online meeting (like GoToMeeting) with a factory that makes molded handles for the new surgical instrument that I'm working on and figure out why the handles aren't fitting properly. Then I go down to the machine shop to pick up some parts for my project and I spend some time in the lab assembling the parts and conduct some testing to see if they cut tissue properly. I record in a computerized lab notebook, "cutting action far superior to last version!" Suddenly it's 6 or 7 o'clock and I wonder, where did the day go!?

It is also important to "walk the talk" about being an engineer. If you believe in something, you should do something about it. So, I serve as a judge of BME senior projects at Worcester Polytechnic Institute and the University of Connecticut. It is very rewarding to share my nearly 40 years of experience with the eager young people in these programs.

Career Outlook

Biomedical Engineers rank #6 in Best Engineering jobs. The Bureau of Labor Statistics predicts that there will be a 4% increase in biomedical engineering jobs through 2028, with 700 new jobs. Experts consider this job growth to be as fast as the average growth rate for all jobs. The demand for biomedical advances will likely be due to the aging baby boomer population. The median biomedical engineer salary is $88,550, with a 2% unemployment rate. As of July, 2019, the demand for BMEs has increased. Many companies report difficulties in filling BME positions. Experienced BMEs are changing positions to get higher salaries. The demand for BMEs will only increase as the huge wave of "baby boomers" (people born between 1946 and 1964) age and require more medical care. Particular areas of growth include telemedicine (practicing medicine from a distance, e.g., over a 5G network), at-home care products (so aging people can better take care of themselves at home and stay out of institutions), and devices that use artificial intelligence (AI) to diagnose disease earlier so that they can be treated (e.g., behavioral monitors that can detect signs of Alzheimer's Disease even before an individual or their family become aware of symptoms).

Search and Explore

PennState Biomedical Engineering Guide
http://guides.libraries.psu.edu/c.php?g=318448&p=2258484

The IEEE Engineering in Medicine and Biology Society (EMBS), world's largest international biomedical engineer society
https://www.embs.org/

List of the top 40 medical device companies – Medical Device and Diagnostics Industry Published February 19, 2019
http://www.mddionline.com/article/top-40-medical-device-companies

BioPharma Guy Directory of Biotechnology, Pharmaceutical & Medical Device Companies
http://biopharmguy.com/links/company-by-location-medical-devices.php

Best Value Schools, 50 Best Value Schools for Biomedical Engineering 2019
https://www.bestvalueschools.com/rankings/biomedical-engineering-degrees/

2019 Biomedical Engineering / Bioengineering Rankings, US News & World Report
https://www.usnews.com/best-graduate-schools/top-engineering-schools/biomedical-rankings

Videos:

https://www.youtube.com/watch?v=QlnZpv713V4

https://www.youtube.com/watch?v=TkKeO5D_eMI (Bringing sight to the blind)

https://www.youtube.com/watch?v=-GA9gEh1fLs (Bringing hearing to the deaf)

https://www.youtube.com/watch?v=J9PQiWkJCtl (Learning to walk again)

CHAPTER 17

Clinical/Counseling Psychologist

Pamela J Ginsberg, Ph.D.

Education:	Bachelor's Degree (Psychology or related field)	4 years
	Master's Degree (Clinical or Counseling Psychology)	1-2 years
	Doctoral Degree (Clinical or Counseling Psychology)*	3-4 years
	Post-Doctoral Fellowship (optional)	1-2 years
License:	Examination for Professional Practice in Psychology (EPPP)	
	State Exam required in most states	
Median income:	$79,010 (range, $43,800 - $129,250)	

*Doctoral Degree is a Doctor of Philosophy (Ph.D.) or Doctor of Psychology (Psy.D.)

Why I Became a Clinical/Counseling Psychologist

I decided to become a psychologist when I was about eight years old. I was watching a TV show which featured a psychiatrist, and I was intrigued and fascinated about the idea of talking with people about their problems and helping solve them. As I grew up, I learned as much as I could about a career in psychology. By the time I went to college, I was sure that I would pursue a doctoral degree and be a psychologist. During my training, I struggled to find an area of specialization that I really loved. I experimented with several specialties including marriage and family therapy, teaching in a university setting, women's issues and health psychology. I finally found my passion in oncology. I work with cancer patients and their families in a private practice setting. I also do quite a bit of public speaking for various local and national cancer organizations to help educate patients and healthcare providers about the psychological health and healing of cancer patients and their caregivers. I am affiliated with my local hospital and cancer center and I serve on a board of directors for a large cancer organization that provides social and emotional support for cancer patients and families. I have owned my private practice/consulting business for over 20 years.

Overview

Psychology is a very broad profession with hundreds of areas of specialization and employment settings. The American Psychological Association has 54 Divisions, which are areas of interest and sub-disciplines. Some of these include: school psychology, military psychology, adult development and aging and developmental psychology. You can find more divisions on the American Psychological Association's website (see references). In this chapter, I am going to focus on the areas of Clinical and Counseling Psychology.

Clinical and Counseling Psychology are quite similar to each other. Clinical psychology focuses on mental disorders and more severe psychological problems, although the psychologist also can treat less severe disorders. Counseling psychologists focus on emotional, social, work-related and physical health issues, with a focus on practicing psychotherapy to help resolve these issues.

The clinical/counseling psychologist helps people with mental (or mind), emotional, and behavioral disorders and problems. We focus on research and practice. Psychological research informs psychologists about intervention approaches or plans. We apply scientific principles to develop and apply different treatment plans. Psychologists use psychotherapy (counseling) to help people overcome problems with everyday life, emotional disorders like depression and anxiety, and problems in their important relationships.

Clinical/counseling psychologists help people with severe psychological disorders such as schizophrenia, as well as less severe disorders such as depression or anxiety. We also see people who are having life problems that do not represent a psychological disorder, such as marital or family problems, health related issues such as cancer or diabetes and life stressors such as losing your job or the death of a loved one. We help people with career decision making, managing stress, losing weight and quitting smoking, school related problems and many other things. Psychologists treat people from early childhood to old age, although many psychologists specialize in a certain age range (such as children or geriatrics). Psychologists treat people of every race and ethnic background and are trained to be sensitive and aware of multi-cultural issues and how they affect a person's emotional health. Psychologists also treat males, females and transgendered people.

The responsibilities of the clinical/counseling psychologist are varied. For those of us who work in direct service professions, we are responsible for client confidentiality, keeping accurate and complete records, billing insurance companies, diagnosis (which often includes psychological testing) and treatment. We must carefully schedule our clients and provide a safe and comfortable setting for them. We are required to use evidence-based interventions (based in sound psychological research) to help our patients (sometimes we call them our clients) overcome their problems and challenges with which they are concerned. We also are responsible to stay well educated and keep ourselves updated about developments in the field of psychology and we regularly attend educational programs to help us with that. We often communicate with other health professionals who may be involved in a client's care.

Specialties and Subspecialties

There are many specialties and subspecialties within the field of psychology, and even within the field of clinical/counseling psychology. For example, my subspecialty is a field called psycho-oncology, which is working with the psychological health of cancer patients. Clinical/counseling psychologists may be specialists in any of the following: teaching of psychology, developmental psychology, school psychology, military psychology, geriatric psychology, rehabilitation psychology, sports psychology, substance abuse, hypnosis, trauma, child psychology, health psychology, neuropsychology, forensic psychology or gender issues. This is just a sample of the many areas of sub-specialization within this field. For even more sub-specialization areas and some descriptions of them, visit the American Psychological Association's website at http://www.apa.org/about/division/index.aspx?tab=2.

In addition to the many areas of specialization, there are also many work settings in which a psychologist may be employed. These include private practice, hospitals, psychiatric facilities, community mental health centers, universities and colleges, college counseling centers, medical practices like doctor's offices, government agencies, businesses, schools and VA centers. Some non-traditional settings include major sports organizations, legal settings, political settings and medical schools.

Requirements

To be admitted to graduate school in clinical or counseling psychology, you must have an undergraduate degree in psychology or a related field, such as social work, sociology or other life sciences. Required classes include basic psychology, abnormal psychology, developmental psychology, statistics, memory and cognition, research and other related classes. Most undergraduate psychology programs also include an internship, which is very helpful for admission into graduate school. Admission into graduate school often requires you to take the GRE, the additional psychology subtest and have an onsite interview.

Graduate programs in counseling and clinical psychology are plentiful across the country. The American Psychological Association (APA) accredits many of these programs and the profession recommends that you attend an APA accredited program, as it makes licensing in most states easier once you graduate. You can earn either a Ph.D. or a Psy.D. degree. They are similar to each other, with the Ph.D. slightly more research focused, while the Psy.D. is slightly more practice focused. Both degrees require completing a doctoral internship and a doctoral dissertation. In most cases, it takes four to six years to complete graduate school, which includes earning a master's degree. In my case, it took me two years to earn my master's degree and four years to earn my Ph.D. degree in counseling psychology, which included the full year of internship.

In graduate school, you are expected to take courses in a wide variety of topics and you can choose an area of study as a specialization. I will describe some of these specializations later in this chapter. Graduate school is a combination of taking classes, engaging in research, accruing considerable hands on experience with patients and often working closely with professors in various projects. During my graduate school experience, I was awarded a "fellowship" which involved teaching undergraduate and graduate classes, conducting research with my professors and working as an editorial assistant for a professional counseling psychology journal. This fellowship helped me to pay for graduate school while obtaining invaluable experience.

The doctoral dissertation is one of the most daunting aspects of earning a doctoral degree. The dissertation is a large research project, which the graduate student designs and carries out. There is a great deal of assistance from professors and you begin working on the dissertation at least by the program's second year. Although it is a bit scary to think about, I found the dissertation experience to be rewarding and interesting. Comprehensive exams are also a requirement in most doctoral programs (sometimes called "comps") and they are a test of all the knowledge you have gained in graduate school in your required academic areas.

Once you graduate, you must be licensed to be a practicing psychologist. You must pass the national licensing exam, which is called the Examination for Professional Practice in Psychology (EPPP) and most states also require that you pass a state exam. Many states require a year of supervised practice before you are able to sit for the licensing exam. Many people take advantage of postdoctoral fellowships for a year or two to obtain the supervised practice and they learn advanced training in a particular area of specialization.

A Day in the Life of a Clinical/Counseling Psychologist

My typical day starts early, often with a business networking meeting as early as 7:00 am. I see patients in my office most of the day, often seeing as many as nine or ten patients, and often working until 8:00 pm. I also travel to other locations to run support groups, attend meetings or consult with others. I present some form of educational or public speaking program about once a month. I am also responsible for all the administrative duties of running a business, such as bookkeeping, managing any technology problems, maintaining office supplies and advertising. I love my chosen career. It is deeply gratifying to me to help people during a time of crisis and see them grow and learn to manage their lives more effectively. Sometimes it is very challenging and emotional, but it brings a sense of meaning and purpose to my life that keeps me going.

Career Outlook

According to the U.S. News & World Report, psychologists rank #39 in the 100 Best Jobs, and #1 in Best Science Jobs. Psychologists earn a median income of $79,010, with an unemployment rate of 0.9%. It is expected that between now and 2028, there will be 26,100 new jobs. Most recently, healthcare has become more accessible to more people which is helping to increase the demand for more psychologists as the population ages. In addition, School Psychologists are ranked #45 in the 100 Best Jobs and #2 in the Best Social Service Jobs. School Psychologists make an average of $76,990 (range, $56,560 - $120,320), with a 0.9% unemployment rate, and a 15% job growth rate creating 23,800 new jobs for school psychologists through 2028. According to data from the National Science Foundation's 2015 National Survey of College Graduates (NSCG) to analyze salaries for psychologists, 2015 Salaries for Psychologists

Executive Summary, the average salary of a Ph.D. psychologist was $85,000, and the average salary of a Psy.D. psychologist was $75,000. It is important to realize that salaries for clinical/counseling psychologists vary widely based on experience, work setting and areas of specialization.

Search and Explore

The American Psychological Association (APA)
http://www.apa.org

The APA Division for Clinical Psychology
http://www.apa.org/about/division/div12.aspx

The APA Society of Counseling Psychologists
http://www.div17.org/
http://www.apa.org/about/division/div17.aspx

The American Counseling Association
https://www.counseling.org/about-us/about-aca

The Association for Psychological Science
http://www.psychologicalscience.orggs

Similar Careers

Recreational Therapist

Social Worker

CHAPTER 18

Physical Therapist

Michael Lazara, PT, DPT

Education:	Bachelor's Degree	4 years
	Doctor of Physical Therapy (DPT)	3 years
	OR	
	Pre-Physical Therapy Undergraduate	3 years
	Doctor of Physical Therapy (DPT)	3 years
	(Only certain schools offer this second option.)	
Certification:	National Physical Therapy Exam (NPTE)	
Optional:	Board-Certified Clinical Specialist (≥ 2,000 clinical hours)	
Median Income:	$87,930 (range, $60,390 - $123,350)	

Why I Became a Physical Therapist

As a child, I always loved sports. In grade school, I played basketball, baseball and tennis. This meant I would also have my share of sports-related injuries. When I was 11, I remember having knee soreness while playing basketball. Then I was diagnosed with a condition called Osgood-Schlatter's a disease that causes pain and inflammation below the kneecap. This disease affects children during their growth spurt. When I was 16, I landed on my hand during a basketball game and broke my wrist. While my wrist was still healing, I decided to continue playing tennis with a cast on. This was probably not the best decision. As a freshman in college, I would go to the gym. I hated that I could not engage in certain exercises because of intense shoulder pain. I eventually self-diagnosed rotator cuff tendinitis.

As I began school at The College at Brockport in upstate New York, I was still undecided on my major. I initially thought that I would study finance like my dad. However, I really enjoyed sports and fitness, which led me to choosing exercise physiology as my major. After speaking with my advisor about future job options, I began to realize that I would need more than a bachelor's degree in exercise physiology to obtain a job that would pay well. I then considered physical therapy as a major. My introduction to physical therapy was at a local outpatient orthopedic clinic near my home in the greater Syracuse, New York area. The clinic was where my grandmother periodically attended for several years after a failed back surgery left her using a walker. I observed one of their therapists treating patients who had a similar condition to the sports-related injuries that I had suffered from while growing up. I began to wonder how much faster my rehabilitation would have been had I known about physical therapy at that time. Over the next few months, I volunteered in different practice settings and finally decided to become a physical therapist (PT). I am grateful to have made the right choice in choosing this career. I feel very lucky and honored to be one of the people in this world who can say that for a living, they help people.

Overview

As a PT, the goals are to help patients decrease pain and regain function and mobility through treatments other than medication and surgery. When a patient first visits a PT, the PT completes an evaluation with a goal of finding any specific problems related to movement and imbalance. Subsequently, the PT develops an appropriate care plan for each patient. This plan may include a combination of strengthening, stretching and manual therapies based on a patient's ability to perform these activities. The plan is designed to return the patient to his or her maximum level of functioning and mobility. Physical therapists are trained in many different types of manual therapies, some of which include: soft tissue massage, trigger point/myofascial release, joint mobilization and manual stretching. PTs work with patients of all ages, from newborns to older individuals. This includes patients who may be in a nursing home or hospital, due to a debilitating medical condition that caused difficulty performing everyday tasks (e.g., walking). The PT's responsibility is to examine patients, diagnose the issue, and then create, implement and adjust a care plan.

Specialties and Subspecialties

There are many different specialties and settings where a PT may choose to work, depending on his or her interest and experience.

Orthopedic Physical Therapy: This focuses primarily on sports related injuries or injuries related to the musculoskeletal system including bones, joints, muscles, ligaments and tendons.

Neurological Physical Therapy: This focuses on rehabilitating patients who have suffered from a neurological condition such as spinal cord injury, stroke, traumatic brain injury, Parkinson's disease, multiple sclerosis or inner ear/balance conditions.

Cardiopulmonary Physical Therapy: This focuses on treating patients with heart and lung conditions such as chronic obstructive pulmonary disease (COPD), cystic fibrosis, heart attacks and other related conditions.

Pediatric Physical Therapy: This focuses on working with children of all ages from infants to adolescents. Therapy focuses on identifying developmental delays and dysfunction due to trauma or genetic conditions. Some examples include cerebral palsy, muscular dystrophy and/or birth defects.

Geriatric Physical Therapy: This focuses on treating older adults with conditions such as arthritis, cancer, osteoporosis, cognitive conditions such as Alzheimer's disease or dementia and treating patients following total knee or hip replacement surgery.

Since PTs serve so many different patient populations, they can practice in many different settings from hospitals to fitness centers.

The acute care setting within a hospital treats recently admitted patients with trauma, severe illness or major surgery. Patients typically stay less than a week in the hospital, and PT follow-up is in a rehabilitation clinic or in their home. An acute care PT may be a generalist or a specialist but will often treat a wide range of conditions including post-operative orthopedic, neurological, general medicine, cardiopulmonary and cancer.

Some other practice settings include: outpatient clinics/offices, physician offices, inpatient rehabilitation facilities, fitness centers or sports training centers, schools, education or research centers, homes, hospices, workplace or occupational environments, skilled nursing facilities, extended care facilities or subacute rehabilitation facilities. Outpatient clinics/offices usually serve patients with orthopedic, sports or musculoskeletal needs such as an ankle sprain or knee injury. For patients who have undergone surgery, outpatient PT is typically the last phase of rehabilitation that bridges the gap between the hospital and the gym. Outpatient clinics typically treat higher functioning patients who can travel back and forth to the clinic on their own. Treatment at home is an option for patients who are homebound or cannot travel to an outpatient facility. Depending on a patient's condition or injury, a PT session typically lasts for about an hour, two to three times a week over a defined period. Some patients may require more intensive rehabilitation to improve their overall mobility and function, with therapy for at least three hours, five to seven days a week (this therapy session might also include speech and occupational therapy). Treatment would then take place in a rehabilitation clinic/hospital. These facilities are often within, or connected to a hospital. Subacute rehabilitation occurs in a special hospital setting where staff provide medical and rehabilitation care to patients who require assistance with daily living activities (ADLs) such as eating, getting dressed and using the bathroom. These patients may see a PT for one or two hours, three to five days a week, where the sessions are not as intense or as long as they are in a rehabilitation (rehab) hospital or acute care setting. Some examples of patients who receive treatment in an acute- or sub-acute facility include those who have had a stroke, a recent total knee replacement or a total hip replacement. These patients may not be ready to go home and usually stay in a subacute rehab facility prior to transitioning to home. Then, they may continue PT with a home care therapist or at an outpatient orthopedic or neurological rehab facility, if necessary. A skilled nursing facility or long-term care/extended care facility typically treats older individuals with musculoskeletal or neuromuscular conditions who would benefit from therapy to maximize function. Physical Therapists can also work for performing arts companies (e.g., like dance companies, theater companies, traveling ice skating/shows), sports teams and sports organizations.

Requirements

Physical therapy is a doctorate program (DPT). To be admitted into a DPT program, you must fulfill certain prerequisite class requirements that you usually achieve through a four year undergraduate degree. Think about what your undergraduate major will be if you are considering becoming a physical therapist. This will help you complete the required prerequisite courses for your application to DPT school, as well as fulfilling your school's major and degree requirements. The most common undergraduate majors applying to PT programs are biology, exercise science, kinesiology, athletic training and psychology. Required prerequisite classes normally include anatomy and physiology and their associated labs, physiology, biology, general chemistry and lab, general physics and lab, psychology and statistics. You can find other specific program requirements on the Physical Therapy Centralized Application (PTCAS) website (see references). In addition, when applying for DPT programs, applicants must have PT experience (with a Physical Therapist verifying the hours), letters of recommendation and GRE scores. Some schools may require an interview.

Most DPT programs participate in PTCAS; however, 25 programs do not. Students wishing to apply to a non-PTCAS program need to apply directly to the institution through its application site. It is extremely important that if you are interested in becoming a physical therapist that you attend a DPT program that is *Commission on Accreditation in Physical Therapy Education* (CAPTE) accredited. You will only be able to take the National Physical Therapy Exam (NPTE) if you have graduated from a CAPTE-accredited program. Currently 233 DPT programs are CAPTE accredited.

The DPT is a relatively new degree in PT education. The Master of Physical Therapy (MPT) and Master of Science in Physical Therapy (MSPT) degrees are not available to new students. There are still many practicing PTs who do not have the DPT degree. Course content in the DPT program includes some of the following topics: biology/anatomy, cellular histology, physiology, exercise physiology, biomechanics, kinesiology, neuroscience, pharmacology, pathology, behavioral sciences, communication, ethics/values, management sciences, finance, sociology, clinical reasoning, evidence-based practice, cardiovascular and pulmonary, endocrine and metabolic and musculoskeletal systems. Eighty percent of the curriculum is comprised of classroom (didactic) and laboratory learning. The remaining 20% is dedicated to clinical education which is usually seven months.

All PTs must pass the NPTE to obtain a license and practice. The Federation of State Boards of Physical Therapy (FSBPT) administers licensing of physical therapists (http://www.fsbpt.org/ExamCandidates.aspx). Most states require CE for license renewal.

PTs may continue their education and receive Specialist Board Certification. This requires at least 2,000 additional clinical hours in the specialization area. There are currently eight areas of PT specialty certification: Cardiovascular and Pulmonary, Clinical Electrophysiology, Geriatrics, Neurology, Oncology (cancer), Orthopedics, Pediatrics, Sports and Women's Health.

PTs looking to further advance their skills and knowledge post-graduation also have the option to apply to a residency or fellowship program in their respective area of interest or specialty (http://www.abptrfe.org/Home.aspx).

Working as a PT in a busy outpatient office or clinic requires having outstanding multitasking and time management skills. In addition, CE helps in keeping up-to-date with new techniques and practices which are key to surviving a demanding and rewarding health career.

A Day in the Life of a Physical Therapist

I work in an outpatient orthopedic clinic. My day typically starts by reviewing my daily schedule, which usually consists of seeing 14-16 patients. Within this workload are usually one or two initial evaluations (new patients). A physical therapist assistant and a physical therapy aide would review my day with me. After looking at this schedule, I will then go through each patient's flow-sheet to update the exercise program as appropriate, based on: the patient's therapy progress, his or her subjective status which includes current functional ability, pain levels and/or post-operative protocol. Although it is crucial to plan before the day starts, a therapist needs to be able to quickly adjust based on how each patient feels that day. As patients arrive, they usually begin their treatment with a moist hot pack or an active warm-up such as using a stationary bike or an elliptical machine. This promotes increased blood flow prior to beginning their exercise program. As an outpatient physical therapist, I spend much of my time performing different manual techniques with a patient, which I do either before or after a patient completes his or her daily exercises. Manual techniques include soft tissue massage, trigger point release, joint mobilizations, manipulations or manual stretching. I am very fortunate to work in a clinic that provides adequate support staff. I work with PT aides, who are often part-time employees currently in an undergraduate program with aspirations to work in the healthcare field. The job of PT aides primarily involves providing and applying moist hot packs and ice, setting up equipment and cleaning the exercise tables. My company also employs other qualified healthcare professionals such as athletic trainers and physical therapy assistants. Athletic trainers usually have at least a bachelor's degree in athletic training and their main responsibility is to ensure that patients are performing exercises correctly. Athletic trainers also help with other treatment modalities such as electric stimulation, ultrasound or laser therapy. Physical therapy assistants work alongside physical therapists in performing various manual techniques, utilizing modalities and progressing patients within their current plan of care. Physical therapist assistants must obtain an associate's degree (five semesters) from an accredited PT assistant program and pass the national examination for licensing upon graduation.

Physical Therapists in an outpatient orthopedic setting must have outstanding multitasking and time management skills, especially during busy times of the day. For example, I may be performing soft tissue massage on a patient with low back pain, while also keeping an eye on a patient who is recovering from post-operative knee surgery who is performing squats, a patient with neck pain performing stretches and a patient with an ankle sprain performing balance activities. The physical therapist must ensure that each patient is performing their exercises or stretches correctly while also having the ability to quickly adjust a certain exercise that may be causing pain. My day usually ends by documenting each patient's progress and subjective status into an electronic medical record system.

A large part of a successful physical therapist is staying on top of current research and attending CE classes. As a therapist, I highly recommend becoming a member of the American Physical Therapy Association (APTA). This organization increases awareness of PT to the public and within the healthcare system. It also provides up-to-date research to promote evidence-based practice and strengthens its members' clinical expertise.

Career Outlook

U.S. News and World Report ranks PTs as number #16 in Best Health Care jobs, and #20 in the 100 Best Jobs. Due to an aging population, the Bureau of Labor Statistics projects a 22% growth in physical therapists through 2028, with an estimated 54,200 new jobs within the next 10 years and an unemployment rate of 1.2%. The median salary was $87,930 in 2018, with the best-paid physical therapists in the top 25% making $101,790 and the lowest-paid 25% making $71,670.

Search and Explore

The American Physical Therapy Association (APTA)
http://www.APTA.org

APTA information for students
http://www.apta.org/ProspectiveStudents/

Commission on Accreditation in Physical Therapy Education (CAPTE)
http://www.capteonline.org/Home.aspx

American Board of Physical Therapy Specialities (ABPTS)
http://www.abpts.org/home.aspx

Physical Therapy Centralized Application
http://www.ptcas.org/

Similar Careers

Athletic trainers - Undergraduate degree in athletic training

Physical Therapy Aides - High school diploma, the desire to work in the medical field, potentially a stepping stone to decide on a future career as a PTA or PT

Physical Therapy Assistants (PTA) - A two-year associate degree program obtained in a CAPTE accredited program and national licensure examination or certification is required in most states to work as a PTA

Occupational Therapist

Podiatrist

CHAPTER 19

Occupational Therapist

María Serrano-Miranda, OTR/L

Education:	Undergraduate science degree	4 years
	Master's or Doctorate degree	2-4 years
License:	National Board Certification in Occupational Therapy (NBCOT)	
Median income:	$84,270 (range, $55,490 - $120,750)	

Why I Became an Occupational Therapist

I felt like I was drowning in college studying for a different allied heath career. I overheard another student talk about her Occupational Therapy (OT) studies. She spoke about the diversity in the OT field (population, work setting, area of practice) and the potential growth in a career as an OT. She was full of passion and life that I just had to see for myself. The very next day, I waited to speak to the Director of the OT Department at my college to ask her about the OT field. I needed and wanted to see for myself if everything that I heard about the profession was true. I was surprised to learn that it was and is! I know that I look upon this encounter as a blessing in disguise. I found my true calling and have never looked back. I have been fortunate enough to have touched the lives of countless people in my career as an OT, and I hope that I have changed their lives for the better. I have also had the opportunity to work in many different settings, which allowed me to gain knowledge, share experiences and make lifelong friendships.

These are some things that make me thankful and secure in my decision to become an OT. I have guided patients to obtain limb movements following surgery, and after having had a stroke or any neurological impairment. I have shown patients how to re-learn skills ADLs such as: dressing, grooming, feeding, and other self-care needs and transferring themselves to a bed or chair. They are activities that people do on a daily basis that are necessary for self-care, and to maintain their independence. Through OT, I have given patients back their independence, something critical that they had lost in their lives during their injury and illness.

Overview and Specialties

Occupational Therapists (OTs) are healthcare professionals who through different therapies, help people participate in activities they do everyday. OT practitioners enable patients of any age to live life to its fullest by preventing injury, or by living better with a disability, illness, or injury and helping patients to promote health. Therefore, an OT provides services to a wide range of the population from infants to the elderly, using practices that are evidence-based meaning they have scientific proof of helping in a particular setting. An OT intervention could include helping a child with disabilities participate fully in school activities and social activities. It could be helping a person who is recovering from a car accident regain control of fine motor skills in their fingers, or it could be providing support for older adults with physical and memory changes to cope better with daily activities. An OT can work in many different settings that include: hospitals, in a patient's home, assisted living facilities, elementary and other schools, universities, nursing care facilities, private care facilities, research and development centers, psychiatric and substance abuse centers, among others. Occupational Therapists use a "whole body" or holistic approach to focus on modifying the task and/or environment to fit the patient. The patient is also an essential partner in their own therapy.

Requirements

A bachelor's degree and master's degree/doctorate degree is required to become an OT. Ideally, the bachelor's degree should be in a science such as biology, chemistry, kinesiology, psychology or sociology, in order to obtain the necessary science prerequisites to apply for a graduate degree in OT. Some schools offer accelerated programs where there is a combined bachelor and master's degree program. To practice as an OT, you also need to graduate from an accredited program and complete field work. Additionally, you must become licensed in the state where you want to practice by taking and passing the National Board Certification in Occupational Therapy (NBCOT) exam. My credential is the OTR/L which means Occupational Therapist, Registered and Licensed.

An OT has different responsibilities depending on the work setting. General duties of an OT are: performing a chart review, and interviewing and observing the patient in natural activities. This helps to establish a treatment plan with specific goals. An OT may also modify the environment to meet the person's needs, provide an exercise program, recommend adaptive equipment and educate those in close contact with the person to better gain health and wellness. Lastly, I keep documentation on activities, progress and assessment (physical, cognitive, psychosocial, sensory and environmental phases of recovery) and provide information to physicians and other health providers.

A Day in the Life of an Occupational Therapist

My day as an OT begins by reviewing my daily schedule of the children I serve in a public-school setting. I review my schedule to plan treatments according to individual child delays, current skills and accomplishing set goals. Next, I reach out to school staff to review and collaborate treatment sessions. Then, I prepare my treatment room for pull-out sessions for that day. Over the next few hours, I perform supportive academic services to the children who are part of my case-load. Some areas that I address are writing skills/management of classroom tools, sensory needs, strength/movement/posture, ADLs, visual-perceptual-motor skills and academic organization and work habits. Once in the morning and once by the end of each day: I document the time, completed on and students' response to the session. I take a quick lunch break and schedule any evaluations that are pending. Closer to the end of the day, I touch base with parents for any pending issues and attend scheduled meetings. Before the work day is over, I communicate with my colleagues, check my emails and tackle any OT issues that I must address. Before you know it, I'm back at work the next day to see those little faces that I help.

Career Outlook

U.S. News and World Report ranks Occupational Therapists as #11 out of the Best Health Care Jobs, and #13 in the 100 Best Jobs. The need for OTs is expected to increase as baby boomers get older and strive to maintain their physical health and independence. The U.S. Bureau of Labor Statistics reports that this profession will grow by 18% from 2018 and 2028, resulting in about 23,700 more professionals in this field. OTs garner an average salary of $84,270 and have a low unemployment rate of 0.5%.

Search and Explore

National Board for Certification in Occupational Therapy (NBCOT)
http://www.nbcot.org/about-occupational-therapy

Accreditation Council for Occupational Therapy Education (ACOTE)
https://acote.aota.org/

American Occupational Therapy Association (AOTA)
http://www.aota.org/

Similar Careers

Physical Therapist

Occupational Therapist Assistant – Associate's degree from an accredited occupational therapy assistant program.

Occupational Therapist Aide - a high school diploma or equivalent, and on the job training.

Recreational Therapist (Art, Music, Drama)

Social Worker

CHAPTER 20

Social Worker

Suzannah Callaghan, LCSW-R

Education:	Bachelor's Degree	4 years
	Master's Degree (Social Work)	2 years
	Supervised Psychotherapy Practice	3 years
License:	Clinical Social Worker (LSW) or LCSW or LISW or LICSW	
Median income:	$49,470 (range, $30,750 - $81,400)	

Why I Became a Social Worker

I became a social worker because I learned about "the talking cure." When I was a teen, I saw friends and family members speaking to professionals about solving and coping with their problems. I have always enjoyed helping people who are struggling and wanted to find ways to make people's lives brighter and better. In college, I volunteered at a center for domestic violence where I provided hotline support to people whose romantic relationships had become dangerous. I felt proud to be able to create a safe space for people, over the phone, where those in pain could talk about their situations without being judged, and where I could gently offer choices to people who were unsure of where to turn.

Overview

As a Licensed Clinical Social Worker (LCSW), I work with people who are experiencing mental health issues. Some patients have anxiety, where they worry so much that it gets in the way of being able to live and function. Others struggle with depression and get so sad that regular daily life – such as keeping up with work or school – is unmanageable. Some have difficulties with their thoughts or perceptions of what is real. LCSWs can work with people of all ages or work with a specific age group. I work with adults and I provide psychotherapy to them to help them best manage whatever is difficult for them.

LCSWs can work independently, but we all do best when we are meeting with other social workers or mental health professionals to discuss our cases in supervision, which can either be in group settings or in one-on-one settings. Some of us choose one other social worker to talk about our struggles with our patients, and some of us meet in groups to talk about patients and challenges.

Specialties and Practice Settings

Private Practice: LCSWs who work in private practice see patients in a private office. They usually meet with their clients weekly. Many work with individuals and some choose to work with couples, families or offer group therapy to patients. They might work with children or specialize in working with seniors. They may focus their practice on eating disorders or choose to focus on working with mothers with post-partum depression. In this setting, LCSWs set the fee that they charge and can decide whether they want to accept insurance for their services. The LCSW is then responsible for all issues related to billing and dealing with insurance companies (if applicable).

Clinic Setting: LCSWs can work in a mental health clinic. In this setting, the clinic helps them find patients and the clinic sets the fees that the clients pay and gives the LCSW a fee for the clients they see. In this setting, someone else is usually responsible for dealing with billing issues.

Hospital Setting: LCSWs in a hospital setting can work in several different areas. They might work with hospitalized patients, providing therapy to help the patient regain the ability to live independently. They might work in a day-treatment facility, offering group or individual therapy and psychoeducation and activities to patients who need a therapeutic setting during the day – who aren't yet able to maintain a job or go to school - but can live at home. They might also work in a clinic setting, like the ones already described.

Requirements

To practice as a clinical social worker who provides psychotherapy, you first need to obtain a bachelor's degree. I chose to study psychology. This gave me a strong foundation for the classes that I later took while pursuing my master's degree. These classes included studying about human behavior and brain functioning. During the master's degree in social work, I spent about half of my time learning theories and practices in a classroom setting. The other half of my time was working in the field – a field placement – it is like a school-based internship. During field placement, I was able to practice the ideas I was learning in class and I worked with clients/patients under the close supervision of a more experienced social worker. The master's degree in social work was two years. Each year had its own extensive field placement.

After I received my master's degree, I took a licensing exam. This license was my first step towards practicing as a social worker, but I still wasn't yet considered "a clinical social worker" - someone who could independently offer therapy without very close supervision. I received weekly supervision, with my supervisor reviewing my cases with me and helping me best serve the needs that arose for the patients. My supervisor also helped me evaluate any areas where my own biases or issues kept me from helping the patients as best as possible. As a therapist, I find out what is going on with my patients, but also I am able to understand my own issues that arise while working with them. The names of the licensing exams vary from state to state. In New York, the exam to become a licensed clinical social worker is called the LCSW exam. To be licensed to work independently as a clinical therapist, I needed to have three years of weekly supervision and to pass another licensing exam (LCSW). The second licensing exam allows me to move from a licensed master's social worker to a LCSW, which means you have a license to practice as a therapist on your own, without mandatory weekly supervision, and you can work in your own practice rather than in an organization or for someone else.

Like many social workers who want to work as psychotherapists, I also chose to pursue more learning about therapy in a post-master's training program. There are many different therapy methods that help people. A post-master's training program might teach one therapy method in a more in-depth way. For example, the program might teach a type of therapy that helps people who have been through trauma, it might teach mindfulness therapy, or teach trainees to use hypnosis with their patients. Some programs examine how to work with a particular population – such as working with people with eating disorders, or working with people who have been sexually abused or people with substance abuse (drug or alcohol) problems. These programs often offer both classes and close supervision. You can take these in-depth classes while simultaneously working. This is unlike the social work master's degree where most participants are full-time students and not yet able to work in the field.

The requirements and scope of practices of social workers can vary by state. The included websites offer more information about becoming a clinical social worker and different state requirements.

A Day in the Life of a Social Worker

I work in two different settings. During the day, I provide psychotherapy at a psychiatric hospital. When patients are not safely able to live on their own – when they might be at risk of trying to kill or seriously hurt themselves, or they might attack other people because of their mental illnesses, they can come to a hospital for safety. At the hospital, they can receive intensive assistance from a psychotherapist, from therapy groups and from a psychiatrist to help them get back to a more stable and independent living situation. I also help them figure out what is the best place for them once they no longer need the safety of the hospital.

In the evenings, I also maintain a private practice. In my private practice, I see patients who are also struggling with mental illness, but whose issues are not so severe that they need a hospital setting. When I see these patients, I provide weekly therapy to help them best deal with whatever is contributing to their anxiety or depression. Sometimes we explore issues related to their relationships with their families. Sometimes it's their work relationships and sometimes we focus on what is getting in the way of them achieving their life goals. After meeting with these patients, I keep notes so that I can remember the important aspects of our therapy session. For patients who pay with insurance, I also am responsible for submitting bills to their insurance companies. For patients who pay on their own (also known as, out-of-pocket, or self-pay), I write receipts so that they can submit their payments to their insurance companies or so that they can claim the expense on their taxes. Additionally, when needed and when the patient grants me permission, I also speak with other providers about their care. For example, if a doctor is prescribing a medication to the patient which might be impacting their mental health - for example, a birth control pill that is contributing to depression or an anti-depressant to help them with symptoms of depression - I collaborate with his or her doctors to keep them informed about the impact of the medication on my patient, based on my observations in their therapy session(s).

Career Outlook

U.S. News and World Report ranks Clinical Social Worker as #11 in Best Social Service jobs and #83 in The 100 Best Jobs. The median salary according to the Bureau of Labor Statistics is $49,470, the salary range is $30,750 - $81,400, metropolitan areas of California pay the best. The Bureau of Labor Statistics expects a 11% increase in employment by 2028, mostly due to care for the aging baby boomer generation. Approximately 81,200 new jobs are projected to be available, with a 4.5% unemployment rate.

Search and Explore

A Quick Guide, How to Become a Social Worker
http://www.socialworkguide.org/

Social work license requirements
http://www.socialworklicensure.org/

National Association of Social Workers
http://www.naswdc.org/

Similar Careers

Clinical/Counseling Psychologist

Recreational Therapist

Marriage Therapist

School and Career Counselor

Sociologist

Survey Researchers

Substance Abuse, Behavioral Disorder, and Mental Health Counselors

CHAPTER 21

Music Therapist

Rachel N Schwartz, MA, MT-BC, LCAT, CASAC

Education:	Bachelor's Degree	4 years
	Master's Degree	2 - 2.5 years
	Doctoral Degree (optional)	2 - 3 years
	Fellowship (optional)	0 - 4 years
Board Certification:	Music Therapy Board Certification (MT-BC)	
Median income:	$23,000 - $200,000	

Why I Became a Music Therapist

I started going to verbal therapy in my teenage years where I became increasingly interested in the human experience. In conjunction with this, I was also very interested in music. Growing up, I played many instruments: guitar, piano, flute and piccolo. In addition, I sang and participated in high school band and orchestra, and was involved in music events at school. Music allowed me to better connect with others and express myself. Music helped me decompress and find relief from difficult emotions and experiences, and to better understand myself. I found out about the field of Music Therapy from a friend who was seeing a private Music Therapist.

Overview

Music is a primal and deeply expressive form of communication. It serves to connect our feelings, which may not always be as easily accessible through words. According to the American Music Therapy Association, "Music Therapy is the clinical and evidence-based use of music interventions to accomplish individualized goals within a therapeutic relationship by a credentialed professional who has completed an approved music therapy program." One can practice it through improvisation, song writing, singing, toning, music listening, performing, recording, music relaxation, sound baths, using behavioral models and many other musical forms of expression and connection. I work in inpatient psychiatry, and private practice. Through this modality, I assist clients in processing what they experience in the music to help them gain insight into their emotional states, mental health, relationships, behaviors and work towards mental health goals. A music therapist can serve many populations through different forms of music therapy.

Training Specialties

Some therapists have post-graduate training in the specific populations they serve.

Some examples of Music Therapy Specialties include:

Nordoff-Robbins Music Therapist (NRMT): A three level training program with the pre-requisite of five years of clinical Music Therapy experience. This therapy originated in the United Kingdom serving people with various types of disabilities, but is well known for its work with patients with Autism Spectrum Disorder. This is based on the music improvisation model.

Neuro-Music Therapy (NMT): A four-day, 30 hour workshop with a written exam, followed by a fellowship. NMT then allows one to practice in research-based treatment. It is based on using music to address non-musical goals. The most common patients are those with neurological dysfunction.

The Bonny Method of Guided Imagery and Music (GIM): This is a three level training with advanced modules developed by Helen L. Bonny. This is a form of music-assisted therapy that helps the patient connect the conscious to the subconscious. A trained "guide" or "facilitator" selects specific music programs, traditionally classical pieces, to help guide a client or "traveler" through a creative inner exploration.

Austin Vocal Psychotherapy (AVPT): This is a two-year post-master's degree training program based on Dr. Diane Austin's methods of Vocal Psychotherapy. Therapists use this practice in individual treatment focusing on using the voice. Vocal holding and free associative singing are key techniques in this therapy. This method has been successful in helping patients suffering from past trauma.

The Mary Priestly Method of Analytical Music Therapy (AMT): This is an advanced method and four-part training. AMT is a psychodynamic and psychoanalytic approach using music improvisation followed by in-depth processing of the experience through various modalities. Training for this program can take from three and a half to four years to complete.

Licensed Creative Arts Therapist (LCAT): This is a post-master's degree New York State license that Music Therapists, Art Therapists, Dance Movement Therapists, Drama Therapists and Expressive Therapists can all pursue. The LCAT allows these therapists to perform verbal psychotherapy in New York State, and utilize other creative art modalities.

Some therapists have post-graduate training in the specific populations they serve. Some of these include: Autism, Alzheimer's, Pain Management, Neuro-Cognitive Disorders, Neuro-Music Therapy, Group Therapy Training, Psychoanalytic Training, Trauma Training and Child-Life (helping children cope with anxiety, stress, emotional and grief feelings).

Specialties and Subspecialties

Music Therapists work with people across a wide range of populations. Traditionally, Music Therapy serves people with developmental, medical, physical or emotional disabilities. The field has expanded to non-traditional populations, including average people that are looking for something other than purely verbal psychotherapy.

The Music Therapy patient (or client) age can range from newborns to individuals in end-of-life care. For newborns, research indicates that music therapy helps premature infants stabilize their breathing rates. Studies have shown that live music provided by a certified music therapist can increase a premature infant's ability to feed, sleep and self-regulate; whereas, noise can have a negative impact on growth and development. The work can vary from traditional psychotherapy, behavioral therapy and medically focused therapy to transpersonal meditation centered therapy. I work at a hospital on an adult inpatient psychiatric unit. Examples of other hospital departments include the Intensive Care Units (ICUs) including Neonatal Intensive Care Unit (NICU) and Pediatric Intensive Care Unit (PICU), Child Life, Maternity, Oncology, Palliative Care, Epilepsy units and other areas. Some Music Therapists work in private practices. Other sites may include: outpatient care, rehabilitation centers, nursing homes, hospice, neurologic centers, schools, substance abuse programs, homeless shelters, correctional facilities and even yoga studios.

Requirements

There are many paths to becoming a Music Therapist. Some therapists first obtain their Bachelor's Degree in Music Therapy, and then their Master's Degree. A Bachelor's Degree in Music Therapy is not required to obtain a Master's Degree in the field, but one must have studied an approved curriculum in a related field such as music, education, or psychology in order to be considered for a Music Therapy Master's Program. One must also be proficient in voice, guitar, piano and other percussion instruments, as well as have the ability to play harmonies and different repertoires (written music and improvisation). In order to practice as a Music Therapist, one must become a Music Therapist-Board Certified (MT-BC). This is a certification that includes an exam that one takes after receiving a Bachelor's or Master's degree in Music Therapy, completing 1200 clinical training hours, and a supervised internship. Once certified, the Music Therapist must recertify every five years. Within each five year cycle, the Music Therapist must complete CE credits or other professional development.

A Music Therapist is responsible for meeting each patient/client with empathy, patience and support to help them work through their issues.

One must always maintain a code of ethics that the American Music Therapy Association (AMTA) and the (MT-BC) have established. Beyond therapeutic goals, Music Therapists are required to maintain their instruments and keep the therapeutic space safe. If the therapist is part of a treatment team, one must communicate with them by documenting sessions, monitoring patients' progress through treatment goals and objectives, obtaining clinical supervision, seeking out one's own personal therapy and continuing one's education to stay current with licensures, certifications and developments in field.

A Day in the Life of a Music Therapist

I work on an adult in-patient psychiatric unit. These are patients who typically come to the hospital through the emergency department and have been deemed a danger to themselves or others. This population includes people suffering from psychosis, mood disorders, personality disorders, suicidality/ homicidality, substance abuse disorders, behavioral problems, trauma, neurological disorders, as well as other issues or a combination of these disorders.

I begin my day with Interdisciplinary Rounds. These are meetings comprised of the psychiatric team: psychiatrists, resident doctors, nurses, social workers, medical students, psychology interns and the LCATs. Rounds last about two hours where we discuss patient treatments.

After rounds, I write the patient group schedule for the day, which changes according to the patients' needs. There are three to four daily group sessions that I divide with my co-workers (an Art Therapist and a Dance Movement Therapist). I usually do two or three daily groups, each lasting about 45 to 60 minutes. Within the groups, I often practice music improvisation along with verbal therapy and sometimes we utilize songs as an intervention. I also try to make time to see patients for individual sessions. After each group or patient session/interaction, I write an individual note on how each patient presented during the session. In addition, each patient requires an initial evaluation note, a weekly progress note and a discharge note (when they leave the practice). We use these notes to track patients' progress, presentation and attendance in the groups as well as what I observe from the patient within the setting. At the end of the day, I complete my paperwork and group work and I am able to go home.

Search and Explore

The American Music Therapy Association
   http://www.musictherapy.org/

The Certification Board for Music Therapists (CBMT)
   http://www.cbmt.org/

The Association for Music and Imagery
   http://www.ami-bonnymethod.org/

The American Music Therapy Association Students
   http://www.amtas.org/

Similar Careers

Art Therapist

Dance Therapist

Occupational Therapist

Social Worker

Rehabilitation Counselor

Drama Therapist

Expressive Therapist

CHAPTER 22

Art Therapist

Lucia Perez-Kleine, MA, LCAT, ATR-BC, LMHC

Education:	Bachelor's Degree	4 years
	Master's Degree	2 years
Board Certification:	Art Therapy Credentials Board	
License:	(only required in some states)	
Median income:	$55,900 (range, 30,000 to 80,000)	

Why I Became an Art Therapist

I always knew that I wanted to work in a service field. In my life, I had overcome many obstacles and became stronger and more self-aware as a result. I had developed a passion to help others through their self-discovery process and through healing. I also loved being around others. I was fascinated by people and human behavior and believed that I was a creative and patient person. I also have good listening skills. In high school I excelled in art and found "art making" a source of relaxation, personal expression, and focus. I like to think that my artwork functioned as my "visual journal." After one of my art teachers first told me about the art therapy profession, I was immediately intrigued. She said it would be a good fit for me since it combined my favorite subjects which were Art and Psychology. It was the ideal balance of my creative and expressive interests, alongside my interests in the social sciences. I had found my career niche!

Overview

Art therapists are mental health professionals who help patients express themselves through making art and enjoying the life-affirming pleasures that result from the "art making" process. In doing so, they apply human development, psychology and counseling theories and techniques, so that their therapeutic work with patients (or clients) can be healing and life enhancing. Art therapy improves or restores a patient's functioning, as well as heightens his or her sense of well-being. In individual and group art therapy sessions, the art therapist supports patients/clients in their creative process using various art media, including: drawing, painting, sculpting, and collage. Other artistic processes that one can use with patients/clients include photography, video and graphic arts. The art therapist uses the art making process and the resulting artwork to explore and process a patient's feelings, reduce his or her anxiety, improve self-awareness and reality orientation, reconcile emotional conflicts, increase self-esteem, develop social skills and manage behavior and addictions, amongst other goals.

Art Therapy is one discipline of the many creative arts therapies. Other disciplines include Music Therapy, Dance Therapy, and Drama Therapy. Each one requires a different master's degree and board certification in order to work in the respective specialty. Depending on which degree you are interested in pursuing as a career, you can begin preparing in middle or high school by taking courses in art, music, dance, or drama. You should also take social science classes in psychology and sociology.

Specialties and Subspecialties

Art Therapists work in a variety of different settings including hospitals, psychiatric and rehabilitation facilities, wellness centers, prisons and jails, schools, crisis centers, senior communities, private practice, homeless shelters and other clinical and community settings.

Art therapists also work with many different populations including people experiencing developmental, medical, educational and social or psychological impairment. Some art therapists work with veterans and refugees, as well as survivors of trauma resulting from abuse, combat, and natural disaster, while others may work with persons with adverse physical health conditions such as cancer, traumatic brain injury, Parkinson's disease, multiple sclerosis and other health disabilities. Still others, such as I, work with individuals suffering from mental illnesses including autism, dementia, depression, bipolar disorder, and schizophrenia, as well as personality disorders, behavior disorders and substance abuse disorders. Other clients may not be in crisis and may simply wish to seek out an art therapist in a private clinical setting or community center to resolve conflicts, improve interpersonal skills, manage problematic behaviors and addictions, reduce stress and achieve personal insight.

Requirements

To be an art therapist, you must be creative and have a passion for helping others. You also need excellent listening and communication skills, patience, and an interest in human behavior. If you are interested in becoming an Art Therapist, it may be wise to consider schools which offer an undergraduate degree in art therapy or other mental health disciplines. However, these degree programs are rare, so another equally good choice would be to major in either Studio Art or Psychology, and minor in the other. If you are really driven, you could even double major in both.

To be admitted into a master's degree program in Art Therapy, you must fulfill certain coursework in both the arts and behavioral/or social sciences. Typically, most programs will expect that you complete multiple courses in the studio arts, such as drawing, painting, ceramics, and sculpture, as well as the required prerequisite psychology courses, including Introduction to Psychology, Abnormal Psychology, Theories of Personality (or Personality Development) and Child Psychology (or Developmental Psychology).

When applying to a master's degree program in Art Therapy you must also show proficiency in basic areas of the visual arts: figurative drawing, painting and clay modeling. Most master's programs will ask you to submit an art portfolio as part of their application process, in addition to providing a resume or curriculum vitae (CV), a personal statement, letters of recommendation and official undergraduate transcripts. Some programs may also request an interview.

Presently, there are 35 accredited art therapy master's degree programs in the U S. Most programs are two years, full-time; focusing on studies in art therapy, with some that combine a specialization in mental health counseling or child therapy, couples' therapy or family therapy. Some states may require that the Art Therapist have additional coursework in counseling and/or family therapy.

In an art therapy program, students usually take courses in art therapy theory; counseling and psychotherapy; ethics and standards of practice; assessment and evaluation; individual, group, and family art therapy techniques; human and creative development; multicultural issues and research methods. Graduate programs also usually include a practicum (a course where you learn by working in the field) and/or an internship that involves gaining supervised experience observing and working with clients or patients in clinical or community settings.

All Art therapists must complete a master's degree in Art Therapy as well as pass the Art Therapy Credentials Board Exam to become registered and board certified. Depending on the state in which you plan to work, you may be required to obtain a license to practice. In some states, workers become licensed as art therapists or creative arts therapists, while other states allow people to work as art therapists if they are licensed in another field, such as professional counseling.

A Day in the Life of an Art Therapist

On the 32-bed inpatient psychiatric hospital setting where I work, the first part of my day typically involves going to treatment team meetings alongside other members of the interdisciplinary healthcare treatment team. The other healthcare team members may include, but are not limited to: psychiatrists, psychologists, social workers, occupational therapists, counselors, other creative arts therapists and nurses. I find these meetings to be very informative and enjoyable, since we get a chance to share perspectives of how each patient on the unit is progressing and evaluate their treatment plans to see if patients require any changes. My role involves sharing how patients cooperate and participate in group therapy sessions, and their overall progress advancement in resolving their initial psychiatric symptoms. These issues are the ones that initially caused the patient to be hospitalized. Sometimes, I also present patient artwork and provide feedback to the treatment team regarding my impressions of the meaning of the work. I always do this in context to what the patient verbally communicated to me about his or her art and its personal meaning to him or her.

Throughout the day, I lead different therapy sessions, averaging between two to four per day, one of which is usually an art psychotherapy group. Considering the unit's needs and the patients' interests at the time, I create a group schedule that will be the most therapeutic for as many patients as possible. Other kinds of therapy sessions I may lead include movement and exercise, coping and recovery, and verbal psychotherapy or talk therapy. In art therapy sessions, I often facilitate Open Studio Groups where patients have an opportunity to make their own decisions and create artwork using materials of their own choosing. At other times, I come prepared with an art directive such as: "Draw how you have been feeling lately," "Paint a place you feel the most safe and relaxed" or "Create a small clay sculpture that represents a personal goal that you have." As you can probably imagine, every day is unique, fun and challenging!

Between sessions, I spend time documenting each patient's participation level, including the progress he or she has made on a daily or weekly basis. I also check with my colleagues to inform them of any important details related to a patient's case that I have learned from them while in the session, or from talking with them on the unit. At the end of my day, when I have written all my clinical notes, completed the therapy sessions and I have cleaned up – I head home.

I also have a small private practice one or two nights a week. I rent space from a small therapy clinic, where I see individual patients. Here I get to work with clients on a more long-term basis, rather than the short-term while they are in the hospital setting. My private practice patients tend to be less often "in crisis," and this allows me to go in more depth into their personal histories and explore deeper feelings.

Career Outlook

The Bureau of Labor Statistics does not collect data on art therapists but they estimate employment and salaries under therapists, all other." In May 2014, there were 11,770 other therapists employed with a median annual wage of $55,900. The American Art Therapy Association has about 5,000 members in the U.S., and its 2013 survey found that most of these art therapists have an annual salary of between $30,000 and $80,000. Under Recreational Therapists (grouped together) the mean wage in May 2018 was $47,860 with a range of $29,580 to $80,990.

Search and Explore

The American Art Therapy Association
  http://www.arttherapy.org

Art Therapy Credentials Board Inc.
  http://www.atcb.org

American Music Therapy Association
  http://www.musictherapy.org

American Dance Therapy Association
  http://www.adta.org

North American Drama Therapy Association
  http://www.nadta.org

Similar Careers

Dance Movement Therapist

Drama Therapist

Music Therapist

Social Worker (career of: Expressive Therapist)

CHAPTER 23

Medical Imaging Technologist

Young Ju Chang BS, R.T. (R)(MR) ARRT, CRT

Education:	Associate's Degree	2 years
	and/or Bachelor's Degree	4 years
	and/or Master's Degree	2 years
Board Certification:	American Registry of Radiologic Technologists (ARRT), or Nuclear Medicine Technology Certification Board (NMTCB), or Joint Review Committee on Educational Programs in Nuclear Medicine Technology (JRCNMT)	
License:	(required in most states)	
Median income:	Radiographer (including CT): $61,670 (range, $40,630 - $86,350)	
	Sonographer (including BS, VS): $73,200 (range, $50,760 - $99,840)	
	Radiation Therapist: $82,330 (range, $56,360 -$124,320)	
	Nuclear Medicine: $78,870 (range, $55,330 - $104,730)	
	MRI Technologist: $72,230 (range, $50,220 - $99180)	
	Interventional Radiologist (CVI/VI): $ 56,850 (range, $29,340 - $93,100)	

Why I Became a Medical Imaging Technologist

Who do you think would take an x-ray (radiograph) of your body, a nurse or a doctor? Maybe neither. I had my first radiograph in high school when I was hit by a car on my way home from school. I landed on my elbow and it hurt immensely. The doctor examined my elbow and ordered a radiograph to ensure it was not broken. When the doctor left, a radiographer came over and introduced himself. He explained that he was there to take radiographs of my elbow and took me into the examination room. It was a poorly lit room furnished with radiograph equipment and a table. I sat on a stool and the radiographer placed a lead shield on my lap. The radiographer placed the radiograph cassette, a tool that captures images of the body part, on the table. He positioned my elbow on the radiograph cassette to obtain the needed images. He then walked behind a lead lined wall and pressed the button to take the image. Afterwards, he processed the radiograph cassette and viewed it on a computer screen to check the image quality. Once the image met with his approval, he sent it to the radiologist (physician). My experience from the accident made me understand there were more people involved in healthcare than just doctors and nurses. It ultimately helped me decide on a career in medical imaging as a radiographer, and later, as a magnetic resonance imaging (MRI) technologist.

Overview

Medical imaging is taking pictures of the body, using special techniques with different types of machines. By looking at these images, healthcare providers can determine patients' health and well-being by seeing what patients' have or do not have in their bodies. The person who takes those images is a technologist, tech for short. Some different types of technologists include X-ray technologists (or radiographers), computed tomography (CT) technologists, sonographers and radiation therapists. These medical imaging techs work in clinics, hospitals, academic centers, research facilities, prisons and in the government and military. Medical professionals use medical imaging to examine all types of patients– from newborn babies to older people.

There are different specialties within the field of medical imaging technology. There are varying ways to take the images. This can range from getting a hand x-ray/radiograph from a radiographer to receiving a whole body scan by a nuclear medicine technologist through a gamma camera.

Specialties and Subspecialties

The table towards the end of this chapter shows a condensed view of the different medical imaging and associated therapy specialties, subspecialties and certifications associated with them. The American Registry of Radiologic Technologists (ARRT) designates the initials after the specialties, subspecialties and the primary path, as well as the ability to cross train into other specialties and subspecialties. If you do not plan to certify with the ARRT, other national certifications have prerequisites and education available on their websites. The five credentials in the primary pathway are Radiography (R), Nuclear Medicine Technology (N), Radiation Therapy (T), Magnetic Resonance Imaging (MR or MRI) and Sonography (S).

Radiography (R) Technologist: In this role, the technologist works broadly with X-ray beams that pass through the body. They are absorbed or scattered which provide a static image that the technologist records for later evaluation. Images mostly include internal organs, soft tissue and bones. The pattern may occur on film or electronically. Examples include: dental images, mammograms (pictures of the breast) or verifying the correct placement of surgical markers before surgery. You can also provide patients with support through the procedure by helping them know what to expect and talking them through the procedure.

Nuclear Medicine (N) Technologist: This technologist works on diagnostic tests to help physicians diagnose and evaluate serious illnesses such as cancer and those related to the heart or body. You will prepare and inject radiopharmaceutical agents (radioactive imaging agents usually in very small quantities) into patients, then capture images using a scanner or specialized camera. You can also provide patients with support through the procedure by helping them know what to expect and talking them through the procedure.

Radiation Therapy (T) Technologist: Radiation Therapy Technologists are part of the team that helps radiation oncologists, or doctors who specialize in radiation therapy administration plan, administer and monitor these treatments and patient responses. Radiation oncologists often prescribe radiation therapy for cancer patients and other conditions. When implementing therapy, you will use special equipment that generates ionizing radiation to administer therapeutic radiation doses.

Magnetic Resonance Imaging (MR or MRI) Technologist: As an MRI technologist, you are responsible for obtaining the best possible images. During an MRI, radiofrequency waves within a magnetic field help make images of body function or body parts. Patients may be in distress or be claustrophobic. You can also provide support to patients by helping them know what to expect and talking them through the procedure.

Sonography (S) Technologist: As a Sonographer or Ultrasound technologist, the equipment you will operate uses nonionizing, high-frequency sound waves to create images of patient's internal organs and tissues.

After you obtain the first credential, you can enhance your skills with one of nine postprimary pathway credentials, which include: Mammography (M), Computed Tomography (CT), Magnetic Resonance Imaging (MR), Bone Densitometry (BD), Cardiac Interventional Radiography (CI), Vascular Interventional Radiography (VI), Sonography (S), Vascular Sonography (VS) and Breast Sonography (BS). The table below this section lists other acronyms that are associated with medical imaging.

Mammography (M): This pertains to obtaining breast images for routine screenings or in patients with breast lumps that are either potentially cancerous or non-cancerous.

Computed Tomographyor or Computerized Tomography (CT) or Computed Axial Tomography (CAT): This noninvasive medical test provides cross-sectional images that represent a "slice" of the person using calculated ionizing radiation.

Bone Densitometry (BD): This pertains to determine bone health through special X-ray images. Healthy bones are essential to activity. As we age, low bone density or osteoporosis can occur. Slight bone loss can also occur. These tests help healthcare providers decide on the best treatment options.

Cardiac Interventional Radiography (CI): A CI technologist assists with minimally invasive, image-guided procedures to help diagnose and treat heart vessel conditions without surgery. CI technologists work with complicated fluoroscopic equipment which produce continuous X-ray images. You might also assist with heart procedures (see glossary) such as angioplasty, stenting (coronary), pacemaker insertion, atrial septal defect (ASD) closure (see glossary) or other cardiac procedures.

Vascular Interventional Radiography (VI): A VI Radiotechnologist works on myriad conditions in nearly every part of the body, except the heart. These include the circulatory, or vascular system, or other organs (eg, liver, kidneys). There may be some exams that both CI and VI technologists can interchange, but for the most part, they are separate subspecialties.

Vascular Sonography (VS): A Vascular Sonographer uses ultrasound machines that produce vein and artery images using high-frequency sound waves. These images show the structure and movement of blood through vessels as well as internal organ movement. Medical practitioners use these tests to diagnose and treat different medical conditions.

Breast Sonography (BS): A breast sonogram is not invasive and does not use radiation. Medical practitioners use this test to follow-up on an abnormal mammogram or abnormal clinical examination. The breast sonogram uses a transducer, a probe that produces sound waves, on a patient's breast to produce the ultrasound images which a physician then reads. A Breast Sonographer might also assist with interventions such as biopsies.

Acronyms	Meaning
ARDMS	American Registry of Diagnostic Medical Sonographers
ARMRIT	American Registry of Magnetic Resonance Imaging Technologists
CBDT™®	Certified Bone Densitometry Technologist
CBRPA	Certification Board of Radiology Practitioners Assistants
RRA	Registered Radiologist Assistants

My initial path to becoming a medical imaging tech was through the military. I prepared by obtaining a specific score on my Armed Service Vocational Aptitude Battery (ASVAB) test to meet the occupational standards for my career. It helped that I already studied biology, chemistry and physics before joining the military. My education in the military was emotionally, physically and mentally challenging. Not only was I studying radiation physics, human anatomy and human physiology, I also participated in military training and leadership. After passing my national certification examination, I was a radiographer until I had the opportunity to learn MR in the hospital where I was working. I earned my training certificate in MR from taking MR classes and cross-training as an MRI tech. I later became a nationally certified MRI tech after passing the ARRT MRI exam.

Requirements

Most technologists, sonographers and radiation therapists are nationally certified. The certification that many have is the ARRT. They may also have another certification, board and/or a state licensure, depending on the state and the tech specialty. Although the ARRT indicates that its certification is voluntary, 37 states use the ARRT to base their state licensure.

To become a technologist, you need either a two-year college degree or a four-year college degree. Nationally recognized certifications and accreditation programs list colleges and universities that are aligned with the educational needs of the medical imaging programs. To obtain ARRT certification, the school must be ARRT-recognized with accreditation programs listed on their website. For nuclear medicine, the school must be recognized by the Nuclear Medicine Technology Certification Board (NMTCB) and from the Joint Review Committee on Educational Programs in Nuclear Medicine Technology (JRCNMT) and/or the Canadian Association of Medical Radiation Technologists (CAMRT). Most national certifications have joint agreements in registering technologists and/or therapists. This means that if you meet the qualifications for one certification, the other will allow you to take its certification examination. You can check for this information on the certification websites that are listed at the end of this section. It is always best to check to ensure that a national certifying body recognizes the academic program that you plan on taking and has national and regional accreditation.

Medical imaging education is not just available in colleges or universities. It is also available in some hospitals and the military. However, there may be prerequisites or requirements needed prior to acceptance and enrollment into these programs. For hospital programs, prerequisites will be listed on the website. For the military, you must be involved in military service to get into one of their programs.

A Day in the Life of a Medical Imaging Technologist

As an MR tech, I review physicians' orders and identify the reason for the exam. I then bring the patient to a screening room and ensure that there is no metal on or implanted inside the patient. Metals that are attracted to the MRI can cause serious harm to anyone since the MR machine is a very strong magnet that will pull metal towards it very quickly. After this screening process, myself, and/or another tech bring the patient into the room and position him or her on the MR table with special equipment called radio frequency (RF) coils. We place these on the patient's body, where the image is needed. I instruct the patient not to move for the entire exam. Next, I move the patient into the center of the MR machine and leave the exam room to go to the computer, behind the glass wall, where I put in the specific parameters to obtain the necessary body images. I use different techniques to determine which body parts need darkening or lightening so the radiologist and other physicians obtain the best image quality. Finally, once the MRI exam is completed, I take the patient out of the exam room.

Modality	Radiography (R)	Computed Tomography (CT)	Magnetic Resonance Imaging (MR)	Bone Densitometry (BD)	Mammography (M)
Primary path?	Yes	No – need (R) first	Yes	No – need (R), (N), or (T) first	No – need (R) first
Possible modality to cross train to from primary path?	(CT), (MR), (M), (CI), (VI), (RRA), (BD), (S), (BS), (VS)	Refer to the primary path taken	(S)	Depends which primary path was taken	Refer to the primary path taken
Degrees and certificates available (Verify with school or certification board)	Associate's Bachelor's	Associate's Bachelor's Certificate	Associate's Bachelor's Certificate	Certificate	Certificate
Possible certifications /licenses available	ARRT (R) State licensing	ARRT (CT) State licensing	ARRT (MR) ARMRIT State licensing	ARRT (BD) CBT®/CBDT® State licensing	ARRT (M) State licensing

Ultrasound (S), (BS), (VS)	Nuclear Medicine (N)	Interventional Radiology (CI), (VI), (CV)	Radiation Therapy (T)	Radiologist Assistant (RRA
Yes for (S); No for (VS), (BS) – need (R), (N), (T), (S) first	Yes	No – need (R) first	Yes	No – need (R) first
(S) Only→ (MR) for (MR), (VS), (BS) – Depends which primary path was taken	(BD), (MR), (S), (CT), (VS)	Refer to the primary path taken	(BD), (MR), (S), (CT), (VS))	Refer to the primary path taken
Associate's Bachelor's Certificate	Associate's Bachelor's Certificate	Certificate	Associate's Bachelor's Certificate	Master's
ARRT (S), (BS) or (VS) ARDMS State licensing	ARRT (N) NMTCB State licensing	ARRT (CI), (VI) and/or (CV) State licensing	ARRT (T) State licensing	ARRT (RRA) CBRPA State licensing

Career Outlook

The 2018 U.S. News and World Report Best Health Care jobs ranks Radiation Therapist Techs at #27. The Bureau of Labor Statistics projects growth in this relatively small field of 9% through 2028 creating 1,600 new jobs, with a current unemployment rate of 3.6%. Medical Sonographer Techs rank #4 in Best Health Care Support Jobs and #35 in Best Jobs, with a median salary of $72,510, a 1.7% unemployment rate and a predicted employment growth of about 19% through 2028, creating 14,200 new jobs. MRI Technologists rank #14 in Best Health Care Support Jobs, and #89 in The 100 Best Jobs with a median salary of $71,670, a 2.2% unemployment rate and a growth rate of 11% new jobs through 2028, creating 4,300 new jobs.

Professional Societies	Websites
American Society of Radiologic Technologists (ASRT)	https://www.asrt.org
Society of Magnetic Resonance Technologists (SMRT)	http://www.ismrm.org/smrt
Society of Nuclear Medicine and Molecular Imaging (SNMMI)	http://www.snmmi.org
International Society of Radiographers & Radiological Technologists (ISRRT)	http://www.isrrt.org/issrt/default.asp
American College of Radiology (ACR)	https://www.acr.org
Radiological Society of North America (RSNA)	http://www.rsna.org
Society of Diagnostic Medical Sonography (SDMS)	http://www.sdms.org
Association of Vascular and Interventional Radiographers (AVIR)	http://www.avir.org
American Society for Therapeutic Radiology and Oncology (ASTRO)	https://www.astro.org/home

Search and Explore

American Registry of Radiologic Technologists (ARRT)
https://www.arrt.org

Joint Review Committee on Education in Radiologic Technology (JRCERT)
http://www.jrcert.org

Nuclear Medicine Testing and Certification Board (NMTCB)
https://www.nmtcb.org

Joint Review Committee on Educational Programs in Nuclear Medicine Technology (JRCNMT)
http://www.jrcnmt.org

American Registry of Magnetic Resonance Imaging Technologists (ARMRIT)
http://www.armrit.org

American Registry of Diagnostic Medical Sonography (ARDMS)
http://www.ardms.org

Joint Review Committee on Education in Diagnostic Medical Sonography (JRC-DMS)
http://www.jrcdms.org

Cardiovascular Credentialing International (CCI)
http://www.cci-online.org

The International Society for Clinical Densitometry (ISCD)
http://www.iscd.org

Commission on Accreditation of Allied Health Education Programs (CAAHEP)
http://www.caahep.org

Similar Careers

Registered Nurse

Phlebotomist

CHAPTER 24

Clinical Laboratory Technologist

Rova Lee-Huang, M.S., CLT

Education:	Bachelor's Degree	4 years
	and/or Master's Degree	2 years
Board Certification:	American Society for Clinical Pathology Certification (preferred)	
License:	varies by state (only required in some states)	
Median income:	$52,330 (range, $29,910 - $80,330)	

Why I Became a Clinical Laboratory Technologist

Growing up, I was always passionate about helping others and knew that one day I would be doing something in healthcare. I had originally enrolled in a pre-med program in college to prepare me for medical school, but as I began volunteering in hospitals, I quickly found that my compassion for others made it difficult for me emotionally to endure direct relationship with patients. I decided to choose a profession that would allow me to help others without direct patient communication. As part of my university curriculum, I had also been doing research in the genetics department and developed a passion for working in a laboratory. In my senior year, I decided that becoming a clinical laboratory technologist would allow me to have a career in a field that was both healthcare and laboratory related.

Overview

A clinical laboratory technologist (CLT) processes and performs tests on patients' specimens. Testing can range anywhere from blood work on a routine annual doctor's visit to something more critical like diagnosing cancer. Some of these tests require the CLT to operate complex machinery or instruments, while others will require more experience with data analysis. The CLT also must perform quality control of reagents and instruments to ensure the accuracy of the reported results. To reduce variables in testing conditions and methods, the CLT must perform all tests exactly as described in Standard Operating Procedures (SOP). For this reason, employers seek candidates who are highly detail oriented. Since the outcome of tests performed by a CLT directly affects patient care, it is important that the CLT complete testing and report results in a timely manner. Each department has designated "turnaround time" goals for each test to ensure that patients receive their results within a reasonable time limit. Therefore, CLTs also must have excellent time management skills.

Specialties and Subspecialties

There are many different places were CLTs can be employed, beginning with many different types of laboratory settings, some of which include: clinical and diagnostic testing on patient samples in a hospital laboratory, in a commercial/ independent laboratory or in a public health facility such as a Department of Health. Hospital laboratories provide laboratory testing services for specimens from hospitalized (in-house) patients as well as specimens from off-site clinics or medical centers. These laboratories generally are open 24 hours a day. Independent laboratories receive samples/specimens from healthcare facilities that outsource their laboratory testing. Laboratories at the Department of Health perform similar testing, but also monitor public health situations such as epidemics and chemical or bioterrorism threats.

Common subspecialty areas where CLTs can work include: blood banks, chemistry, cytogenetics, cytology, flow cytometry, hematology, histology, immunology, microbiology, molecular pathology and toxicology (see listing below). A generalist is a technologist who can rotate between multiple areas in the laboratory. Becoming highly specialized in any of these areas improves career advancement opportunities to positions such as lead technologist, technical specialist, supervisor or laboratory manager.

Blood Bank: CLTs collect and process blood from donors, identify blood types and blood antibodies, test blood for viruses from blood transfusions and investigate reasons for a patient's rejection response from blood transfusions.

Chemistry: CLTs test for chemical components of blood, such as blood glucose, electrolytes and enzymes that are released into the blood in response to organ damage.

Cytogenetics: CLTs investigate the number and structure of human chromosomes and look for abnormalities to identify genetic disorders. Changes to chromosomal structure can cause gene failure. CLTs commonly perform cytogenetics testing on pregnant women to rule out chromosomal abnormalities in a fetus that may indicate the presence of growth developmental issues. CLTs also can perform cytogenetics testing on oncology specimens to identify chromosomal abnormalities in lymphoma, leukemia and some solid tumors.

Cytology: CLTs prepare patients' samples (e.g., bodily fluids or tissue samples) and stain them on slides for the pathologist to examine under a microscope to determine if any cellular abnormalities are visible.

Flow Cytometry: CLTs use a special instrument that uses laser technology to count individual cell properties. The Flow Cytometer quantitates properties such as cell size, cell surface receptors, cell proteins, DNA and RNA. Medical practitioners most often perform flow cytometry to identify blood cancers.

Hematology: CLTs specialize in testing samples for blood-related diseases. The CLT evaluates blood properties such as white and red blood cell counts, platelets counts, the hematocrit, red blood cell volume and the hemoglobin concentration, to identify blood disorders.

Histology: CLTs work with whole tissues (large areas) or biopsies (small areas of tissue that may appear to be or have the potential to be diseased) that are fixed and prepared on slides for pathologists to examine for abnormalities. Specialists use the results from histology to determine if a tumor is cancerous, and to identify the cancer stage.

Immunology/Serology: CLTs perform testing on serum collected from blood samples to identify infections or disorders in the immune system that can cause self immunity disruption, cancer and other chronic diseases. The CLT also can perform blood titers to determine if a patient has immunity to certain diseases (e.g., varicella, measles, mumps, rubella and hepatitis).

Microbiology: CLTs prepare samples (e.g., bodily fluids, tissue or swabbed samples) and prepare cultures to help identify patient infections. Technologists preliminarily can identify the organism by preparing slides for microscopic examination. The CLT processes patients' samples to help identify the best possible treatment.

Molecular Pathology: CLTs investigate the molecular pathways of diseases and identify disease causing genetic mutations in patients' specimens. Identifying specific mutations and understanding their role in the molecular pathway can help choose the better targeted therapy to maximize treatment efficiency. One can perform molecular testing on extracted microbial DNA (e.g., DNA from bacteria or viruses) to identify a suitable antimicrobial for treating an infection. One also can perform molecular testing on a patients' DNA to identify a cancer causing abnormality or an inheritable disease.

Requirements

High school students interested in pursuing a career in the medical laboratory sciences should take chemistry, biology and math classes. A bachelor's degree in Medical Technology or life sciences is usually required for an entry-level technologist job.

An associate's degree in clinical laboratory science is usually required to become a Medical Laboratory Technician. Military and vocational or technical schools also may offer certificate programs for medical laboratory technicians.

Students interested in becoming a CLT must first complete the requirements for a bachelor's degree in clinical laboratory sciences, medical technology or another related field. Colleges or universities offering a four-year medical technology program will prepare students in all areas of a clinical laboratory setting including coursework and internships. The curriculum consists of chemistry, biology, statistics and math. High school students who are interested in pursuing a career as a CLT can prepare for their academic requirements by choosing more advanced high school courses in math and science (e.g., AP Biology, AP Chemistry, AP Calculus). College students majoring in other sciences but not enrolled in a four-year medical technology program may be eligible to apply for a medical technology program. Once students have completed the program, they must pass the state required exam(s) to earn the proper licensure or certification for employment. The requirements for exam(s) and licensure differ by state. Alternatively, students can complete a two-year program for an associate's degree in clinical laboratory science and then take the required exam(s) to become a laboratory technician. Working as a laboratory technician gives students laboratory experience before continuing on to a four-year CLT program.

A Day in the Life of a Clinical Laboratory Technologist

A typical day usually starts with laboratory maintenance to ensure that all of the equipment is working properly. If the department runs 24 hours a day, seven days a week, there will be a few minutes where the prior shift communicates and hands off the work to the next shift. The CLT receives specimens and logs them. A technologist then processes the sample and performs the test. An example of a test would be examining some lung tissue for the presence of abnormal cancer cells. Each department consists of different areas or tasks which management assigns to technologists and they rotate according to a schedule. This ensures that every CLT in that department is fully competent in all areas of his or her laboratory. CLTs perform tests based on priority and must complete them within the established "turnaround times." CLTs need to perform immediately tests labeled as STAT (which means immediately or emergently). One must enter results in a timely manner so that either the department chief or director can review them. Once reviewed, the designated person immediately reports the critical values that have the greatest impact on the patient's care to the physician.

Career Outlook

According to the 2019 U.S. News and World Report Best Health Care Support Jobs, CLT ranks #1. They also rank CLT as #21 in The 100 Best Jobs. The Bureau of Labor Statistics projects 11% in CLT employment growth through 2028, adding 35,100 more professionals to the current field.

Search and Explore

American Society for Clinical Laboratory Science (ASCLS)
  http://www.ascls.org/

Association for Molecular Pathology
  https://www.amp.org/

American Society for Clinical Pathology
  https://www.ascp.org/content

The National Accrediting Agency for Clinical Laboratory Sciences (NAACLS)
  https://www.naacls.org/

American Society of Cytopathology
  https://www.cytopathology.org/

The Health Department Website for each specific state

Similar careers

Medical/clinical laboratory technician - Associate's Degree or a Postsecondary Certificate. Some states require technicians to be licensed.

Biological Technician - Bachelor's Degree

Chemical Technician - Associate's Degree

CHAPTER 25

Speech-Language Pathologist

Lauren B. Schwartz M.A., CCC-SLP

Education:	Bachelor's Degree	4 years
	and Master's Degree	2 years
	Clinical Fellowship	1 year
	Doctoral degree (optional)	2-3 years
License:	Through a state licensing authority	
Median Income:	$77,510 (range, $48,690 - $120,060)	

Why I Became a Speech-Language Pathologist

When I was in elementary school, my mother had a friend who worked in my school. She would come into my room from time to time, talk to my teacher and take some students out of the room. I wasn't sure at the time why, but I did know that I was intrigued.

It wasn't until my junior year of high school, when starting the college and career search, that I looked back and thought about the idea of becoming a speech-language pathologist. Ever since playing 'teacher' with my friends and with our dolls during our young school days, I had always known that

I wanted to work with kids in some capacity. However, there were also many times I overheard 'horror' stories from some of my mother's friends who were teachers trying to control 20-30 kids all day in their classrooms. I wasn't sure if becoming a classroom teacher was for me. Reflecting back, I remembered my mother's friend from when I was in elementary school, and my curiosity in her profession (speech-language pathology) grew. I contacted her and spoke with her about her career in speech-language pathology. After our conversation, I knew it was a profession I would love to pursue. Knowing that you can help someone gain his or her voice is something that truly fascinated me, and from there my search began for colleges to learn this profession.

Overview

A speech-language pathologist (SLP), sometimes called a speech therapist, is a professional trained in evaluating and treating patients who have difficulties related to speech, language, cognitive or social communication or swallowing disorders. These problems could result from a variety of causes, such as developmental delay, stroke, brain injury, hearing loss, autism, cleft lip/palate or other syndromes. Once the SLP formally evaluates and identifies a disorder or difficulty in an individual, he or she determines the frequency an individual should receive therapy. The SLP devises and implements an individualized treatment program. The SLP reviews and revises the patient's program and goals as needed. The SLP either may provide speech-language services individually or within small groups, which can be with others of similar age and/or disorders, depending on the severity of the diagnosis.

Common speech disorders that SLPs treat are Articulation, the way we say our sounds; Phonology, the speech patterns we use; Apraxia, difficulty planning and coordinating the movements we need to make speech sounds; Fluency, stuttering; and/or problems with the way the voice sounds. Common language disorders that SLPs treat are Receptive language, difficulty understanding language; Expressive language, difficulty using language; and Pragmatic language, the way we socialize and speak to each other. Other common disorders SLPs treat are hearing loss, developing speech or alternative communication systems; Oral-motor disorders, weak tongue, lip or jaw muscles; and/or Swallowing/Feeding disorders, difficulty chewing and/or swallowing.

SLPs serve individuals from birth to adulthood, from diverse linguistic and cultural backgrounds. Some SLPs specialize in working with infants and children and some specialize in working with adults. The range of clients' ages varies by the type of facility. SLPs work in many different settings, most commonly in schools (public and private), day care centers, private practice, clinics, hospitals, rehabilitation centers and nursing homes. Other settings include universities, research laboratories or health agencies.

The decision to work as an educational-based versus medical-based SLP is a common decision to make when deciding your course of study. An educational-based SLP's primary function is working with young children to young adults to improve their social communication, expression and comprehension skills as they relate to daily functioning and academic performance. SLPs typically target their services in the areas of language, articulation/phonology, autism, fluency and feeding. A medical-based SLP characteristically provides evaluations and treatment to individuals with oral-motor, swallowing, cognition and/or speech/language difficulties that have occurred due to medical complications such as stroke, brain injury, cancer, vocal abuse or genetic abnormalities (e.g., cleft lip/palate). These SLPs must also understand medical terminology and procedures.

An SLPs job, in most settings, largely involves direct contact with clients/patients; however, administrative tasks which include ongoing data taking/record keeping, formal and informal testing and progress report writing are also a significant responsibility. In all settings, SLPs must assume various roles in addressing their patient/client needs. Collaboration with families and other professionals is necessary. Other professionals may include teachers, physicians, psychologists, audiologists or occupational and/or physical therapists. To be most effective in an SLP position, one should possess good communication, listening, and critical-thinking skills, compassion, patience and be detail oriented.

Specialties and Subspecialties

Most SLPs are employed by medical centers, hospitals, rehabilitation centers or schools.

School SLPs work in one, several, or many schools. They identify and treat children and are employed by the school system, or potentially by a Health Department, if the school is within their jurisdiction.

Child Language and Language Disorders is a specialty area for those who work primarily with children with language difficulties. These disorders target expressive, receptive, and pragmatic language delays associated with child development academically and socially. Pragmatic language refers to the use of appropriate communication in social situations (knowing what to say, how to say it, and when to say it).

Phonological and Articulation Disorders is another specialty which relates to speech sound disorders. These can be due to neurologic disorders, structural abnormalities (such as cleft palate) and/or sensory/perceptual disorders (e.g. hearing impairment).

Voice / Resonance Disorders includes nasal speech, whereby there is too much or too little nasal and/or oral sound energy in the nasal canal when speaking, or when sound gets trapped in the nasal canal leading to abnormal speech.

Fluency and fluency disorders is another specialty. This pertains to the smoothness, rate and continuity of speech production. Stuttering would be a speech fluency disorder. Stuttering is an interruption in the flow of speaking which often leaves the individual with tension and negative reactions. Cluttering is also a speech fluency disorder. Cluttering is a rapid and irregular speech rate and/or collapsing of syllables. For example, instead of saying "Turn the radio off," the patient says "Turn the radio off." Both children and adults can have fluency disorders.

Swallowing and swallowing disorders are more common in hospitals, health-systems and rehabilitation centers. Here the SLP uses different techniques and instrumentation to determine a patient's swallowing ability. These patients are said to have dysphagia, an inability to swallow and squeeze food down the throat. There are many causes of swallowing disorders. Some are due to nerve or brain damage such as stroke, spinal cord injury, multiple sclerosis, Alzheimer's disease or Parkinson's disease, while some can result from head and neck abnormalities such as throat cancer, bad or missing teeth, mouth or neck surgery.

Aural Rehabilitation specialists work with patients with partial or full hearing loss that occurred early in life or that they acquired some time later.

Requirements

While there is no specific undergraduate major required to become an SLP, the most common major is communication sciences and disorders. If you select another major, prerequisite courses in phonetics, linguistics, language and cognitive development and audiology are typically necessary for admission into an SLP master's program.

A master's degree is the minimum requirement for pursuing a career as an SLP in almost all states. The Council on Academic Accreditation in Audiology and Speech-Language Pathology (CAA) must accredit the selected speech-language pathology master's program. The program generally takes two years to complete and will require up to 400 hours of supervised clinical experience. This consists of 25 hours of clinical observation and 325 hours of direct client/ patient contact. Additionally, most states require speech-language pathologist candidates who want to work with school children to also have a teaching license.

After completing the educational requirements, the SLP student must obtain a passing score on the Praxis exam in speech pathology, as well as complete a 36 week (1260 hours) Clinical Fellowship Year (CFY) in direct clinical practice, to apply for certification in speech-language pathology, through the American Speech-Language and Hearing Association (ASHA).

For those looking to work in research, private practice or as a college professor, it is necessary to earn a doctoral degree. The average time is two to three years beyond the master's degree.

Although voluntary in most states, many employers require the Certificate of Clinical Competence in Speech-Language Pathology (CCC-SLP), which the American Speech Language Hearing Association (ASHA) offers. You can find a complete list of each state's licensing and certification requirements at http://www.asha.org. CE courses are mandated in three-year intervals to maintain your certification and stay current on the latest knowledge and methods related to the field.

A Day in the Life of a Speech-Language Pathologist

Working as a school speech-language pathologist (or speech teacher, as often labeled in school districts), I design and set my weekly schedule at the beginning of the school year. Each day consists of eight 30-minute sessions (a mixture of individual and small group sessions; typically, two to five students each), a 50-minute lunch and a 45-minute preparation/paperwork period. Students in my caseload of 30, kindergarteners to fifth graders, are strategically arranged on my weekly schedule. In collaboration with the teachers, I attempt to schedule sessions so that students do not leave their classrooms during core lessons. I also have to maneuver sessions around lunch periods and other special classes.

My day begins at the start of the first period bell. I visit one to three classrooms and pull out students and bring them back to my room. We sit as a group and complete a chosen lesson/activity, which I design. This targets at least one of each of the students' designated goals set for them in their Individualized Education Plan (IEP). During each lesson, I keep and report data for each student of their performance. After 30 minutes, I walk the students back to their classrooms, with five minutes to travel to one to three more classrooms to gather my next student(s), again bringing them back to my room for their individualized lesson of the day. The morning typically consists of six consecutive sessions, followed by my lunch, then a preparation period. The preparation period is intended to allow me to prepare the next day's lessons; however, I also use it to speak with colleagues to discuss an upcoming meeting, report on students' progress, call parents, or provide advice to teachers concerned about whether they need to refer a student for a speech-language evaluation. The end of my day consists of two more 30-minute sessions, after which the students are dismissed from school. During the final 30 minutes of the day, I input students' progress for that day's sessions into a computerized Special Education Student Information system. The NYC Department of Education has designed this database to aid in monitoring the progress and for Medicaid reimbursement of our students.

Although working in a school setting can be very hectic, due to struggling to catch up on Medicaid paperwork, creating new lessons at home or rushing to screen new students, it is very rewarding. Not only is it an amazing feeling to watch students meet a specific goal, but watching them make progress, grow and develop, is extremely fulfilling. Typically, we work with children (and families) for up to six consecutive years, so we can see them develop over these years.

Career Outlook

According to U.S. News and Word Report, Speech-Language Pathologists rank #18 in Best Health Care jobs, and #23 in The 100 Best Jobs. A pay increase recently occurred in this field where the median salary increased from $66,920 (2010) to $77,510 (2018). There is also a low unemployment rate of 0.8% for SLPs; the best paid 25% of speech-language pathologists made $96,980, while the lowest-paid 25% made $60,200. The Bureau of Labor Statistics predicts 41,900 jobs between now and 2028, sparked by speech and language impairments that increase with aging baby boomers. Analysts also anticipate an increased awareness of speech and language disorders in children to spark this job increase.

Search and Explore

The American Academy of Audiology
https://www.audiology.org/

American Speech-Language-Hearing Association
http://www.asha.org

Council on Academic Accreditation in Audiology and Speech-Language Pathology
https://caa.asha.org/

National Student Speech-Language-Hearing Association (NSSLHA)
https://www.nsslha.org/

American Academy of Private Practice in Speech Pathology and Audiology
https://www.aappspa.org/default

Similar Careers

Audiologist

Social Worker

Psychologist

Recreational Therapist

CHAPTER 26

Emergency Medical Technician

Lenny Nathan, B.A., EMT

Education:	EMT	5 months
	Bachelor's degree (optional)	
Median income:	$34,320 (range, $22,760 - $58,640)	

Why I Became an Emergency Medical Technician

After a 30-year career in the broadcast television industry, I retired in 2003 at the age of 50. I did not know what I would do next, but I knew I wanted to play golf and become involved in the community. That led me to my local Ambulance Corps where I initially began volunteering as the "third wheel" of an ambulance crew. This position was simply known as a "helper."

I had always felt that my career in "television," where I oversaw live sports productions, prepared me for the pressures and time constraints that emergency medical professionals faced. Emergency Medical Technicians (EMTs) are under huge pressure because they represent the first line of care for someone who is injured or sick, who call for medical attention when they cannot get themselves to a hospital. Keeping people calm under tremendous pressure was a part of my life for so long that I was able to adapt to the EMT lifestyle very easily.

Overview

It did not take long for me to realize that this was my calling. I fell in love with helping people. In 2005, I began a nine-year career as a volunteer EMT where I attended to about 4,000 ambulance calls. One completes EMT training by taking a 166-hour program over five months. As an EMT, I was the front-line responder for the public who were sick or injured, and who had called 911 for an ambulance. Most ambulance calls are for EMT BLS (Basic Life Support). Calls that required ALS (Advanced Life Support) were those that had severe trauma where we would have to start IV therapy or assist with cardiac emergencies. EMTs are well versed in cardiopulmonary resuscitation (CPR), but the ALS providers, or paramedics, strictly administer medications and IVs. A paramedic is a more advanced EMT.

Most Ambulance Corps have Youth Corps or programs designed for those under the legal age to become an EMT. Many young people do this to earn school credit and many do it to make an inroad into becoming an EMT. I rode on the ambulance purely on a volunteer basis. While doing this, I saw a change occurring in my county. It was becoming increasingly difficult for Ambulance Corps to attract volunteers during daytime hours. To prevent ambulance service interruption, increasingly more counties were turning to paid EMTs. I was not interested in this as a paid position, so in time I decided that this was no longer a position I wanted to keep.

My experience as an EMT also led me to a leadership role as a training officer at the Ambulance Corps, and as a CPR instructor within the American Heart Association (AHA). I was not a fan of the way most CPR sessions were conducted. In 2007, I started my now 12-year-old company – HealthSav LLC, an AHA authorized training center that provides CPR and First Aid Training.

Becoming a CPR instructor turned out to be something that my new volunteer career was designed to utilize. As a layperson coming into the medical field, I related to the process as a layperson. Having been through the process as a CPR/EMT student, I realized that CPR training courses were not taught in an easily understood manner. Therefore, I wanted to provide information in a more thorough way that students would more easily understand. I also wanted people/students to learn the finer points of CPR because it became apparent to me that people vastly misunderstood it – every single person should know at least a simple form of CPR.

My education and degree in marketing clearly prepared me for this entrepreneurial endeavor and I was energized to bring CPR training to the public in a new way. Traditionally, CPR classes required a minimum number of people to attend. This was not a business model, but a way that the volunteer organizations arranged CPR training for the public. I created a unique business model where individuals were able to register for a course, and it would take place even if they were the only ones in the class. My goal was to train as many people as possible, no matter what the class size.

I have been very active within the AHA as a member of their Board of Directors for eight years in our Tri-County region. I also attend numerous conferences throughout the country on matters of heart and CPR care and served as a contributor to many changes that CPR training programs have implemented. For instance, I began very early on in my courses to discuss the difference between a heart attack and cardiac arrest. I did this because I evaluated this misunderstanding to be a factor in why people don't fully understand CPR. Many questioned my methods, but today, the AHA includes this in their training.

I continue to be fascinated by the process of saving lives, and the work we have yet to do includes training the entire population in this effort. For eight years in New York State (NYS), I worked on a bill to make CPR Training mandatory in high schools. In 2016, we saw the first NYS graduating class with all seniors having CPR Training. This bill has now passed in 39 states as of this writing — I could not be prouder of my role in helping to make this happen.. I look forward to many more initiatives that we are trying to implement with the sole purpose of saving lives. More work is required to promote volunteerism and train people in the community to donate time to their local ambulance corps. Whether individuals are in school or retired, they can give more time towards bettering the community in which they live and help save lives.

Specialities and Sub-specialties

Wilderness Emergency Medical Technician (WEMT) or Wilderness EMS: Usually a BLS trained EMT for working in a rural environment.

Tactical Emergency Medical Service (TEMS): An ALS trained EMT who works in an urban environment closely with the law enforcement for tactical work (e.g. missions, triage, operational medicine) when needed.

Community Paramedic (CP-C): ALS trained with competency in mobile integrated healthcare, and expanded EMS services in rural and urban settings, including various healthcare, mental health and housing and service needs.

Critical Care Paramedic (CCP-C): ALS trained critical care paramedics providing patient care in the pre-hospital, inter-hospital and hospital environment.

Flight Paramedic (FP-C): ALS trained and experienced paramedics currently associated with a Flight and/or Critical Care Transport Team(s) can receive certification as a Flight Paramedic.

Tactical Paramedic (TP-C): Is an ALS trained paramedic professional currently providing critical care in the austere and care-under-fire environments. The expectation of a TP-C is knowledge in casualty assessment, stabilization and evacuation in hostile and austere environments, as well as thorough familiarity with tactical principles, triage and operational medicine.

Tactical Responder (TR-C): Is a non-paramedic functioning in a tactical environment (care-under-fire environment). The expectation for a TR-C is knowledge in casualty assessment, stabilization and evacuation in hostile and austere environments, as well as thorough familiarity with tactical principles, triage and operational medicine.

Work Settings

As an EMT you can work for a private ambulance company, for a hospital or health-system or in a town as a paid employee or as a volunteer.

Requirements

To become an EMT or paramedic, you must first have a high school diploma or GED. You need to be CPR certified and take an approved training program in Emergency Medicine Technology. These programs are about five months in length. The EMT training provides considerable practical skills development, as well as learning about emergency scene operations, rescue breathing, shock trauma assessment and IV therapy. It is all aimed at helping you become one of the well-trained heroes who get to serve on the front lines of medical emergencies. When obtaining your EMS certification, there are two different levels of care from which you can choose. These include Basic Life Support (BLS) and Advanced Life Support (ALS). In most states, there are two levels of EMT certification: (1) EMT-Basic and (2) EMT-Paramedic. A few states also include a level between these known as EMT-Intermediate. We generally just refer to EMT-Basic or EMT-Intermediate certification as EMTs or ambulance technicians. We refer to EMT-Paramedic certification as paramedics (or "medics"). EMT-Basics usually undergo about 120 to 150 hours of training; whereas, EMT-Paramedics usually undergo about 1,200 to 1,800 hours of training.

EMT-Paramedics have much more extensive training. They can give injections or start IV lines and administer medications, while EMT-Basics cannot.

A Day in the Life of an EMT

In my region, EMTs are both volunteer and paid. Since I was retired from a successful career and my interest in EMS was to give back to the community, I had always worked as a volunteer EMT. I began, as many do, as a helper or "third wheel" on the ambulance. I quickly fell in love with EMS activities and decided to become an EMT. I received schooling through our county agency and as a volunteer, the state paid for my training. Classes were from September through December with state exams (both practical and cognitive) in late January. Licensing as an EMT is regulated state by state.

As an EMT, I had specific shift assignments that were usually 10-12 hours. During the shift, I was "on call" which meant that I was available at any moment. All town ambulance corps operate through the 911 dispatch system. Many agencies were on the 911 radio and each had their own set of "tones," or sounds to distinguish the agency from others. Many volunteer EMTs may opt to respond from their homes via notification on a two-way radio or sometimes a pager that only goes off to the sound of that agency's tone. Paid EMTs must always be present at the ambulance building when not on a call. Each ambulance must have a crew of at least two with a driver and an EMT. Two EMTs on the crew would usually alternate each call where one would drive and the other would handle the patient (then they would swap responsibilities).

Many factors determined how busy the day would be. These included the community needs and whether the shift was during the day or the night. You never know how many patients you could see in a day – it could literally be either zero, ten or more. Each call would generally take one to two hours depending on the severity and the distance we had to travel to the location and then to the hospital. After each call, we had to decontaminate ("decon") all equipment that we used so that it would be as clean and sanitary as possible for the next person. If we had down time, we would wash the "rig" (ambulance) since large amounts of road dirt would very quickly accumulate due to all the traveled mileage.

Ongoing training is always a very important element for an EMT. Because we do not use all equipment or techniques regularly, we must be prepared at any time should the occasion arise. Training officers at an ambulance corps try to schedule periodic drills to keep the teams sharp and "patient ready." An EMT is prepared for any kind of activity ranging from a cold or flu call, to a gunshot wound or cardiac arrest. All calls require a professional approach to a patient and his or her needs, regardless of severity. Any patient who feels he or she needs an ambulance deserves top treatment throughout the call.

When we received a dispatch call, the crew immediately responds to the dispatch 911 center that they received the call and then again notifies dispatch that they are on the way. They then notify the dispatch when they arrive at their location. Communication is once again set up with dispatch either at the start of patient transport to the hospital and concludes once at the hospital. These times are logged-in and play an important role in evaluating each call for promptness and a community's efficiency (or lack of), in how their ambulance service is doing.

At the hospital, the EMT must complete detailed paperwork to document the recent patient case. This includes recording the logged times, the initial observation of the patient, the description of the stated problem and everything that the EMT and crew did for the patient. The EMT must check blood pressure and pulse (known as vital sign checks) at least three times prior to hospital arrival. Once at the hospital, the patient is in the care of the EMT until the nurse in charge takes the patient care report.

Basic Life Support (BLS) EMTs handle many calls. A Paramedic handles any calls where a patient has a potential heart problem or needs medication intervention that would require ALS. In our county, any 911 medical call sends an ambulance, two police cars, and an ALS unit to the scene. Once the team determines the call needs, they decide if an ALS or BLS crew will accompany the patient to the hospital.

At the end of a shift, an EMT is required to ensure the ambulance is stocked as designated by protocol and the assigned EMT replaces all items to ensure the next crew is fully stocked, sanitized and ready to respond to the next emergency.

Career Outlook

Analysts project growth of EMTs and paramedics to increase by 7% through 2028, faster than the average for all occupations, with 18,700 new jobs. The need for volunteer EMTs and paramedics in smaller metropolitan areas and rural areas will also continue to increase. Car crashes, natural disasters and acts of violence will continue to require EMT's and paramedic's skills. Age-related health emergencies, such as heart attacks and strokes, will increase due to an increase in middle-aged and older adults and this will create an increased demand for EMT and paramedic services.

Search and Explore

The Journal of Emergency Medical Services
http://www.Jems.com

EMT Life LLC
http://www.emtlife.com

National Traffic Highway Safety Administration's Office of EMS
http://www.ems.gov

The National Association of Emergency Medical Technicians
http://www.naemt.org

National Association of Emergency Medical Technicians (NAEMT)'s Expo
http://www.emsworldexpo.com

The National Registry of Emergency Medical Technicians
http://www.nremt.org

The American Heart Association
http://www.heart.org

HealthSav, LLC
http://www.healthsav.com

International Board of Specialty Certification
https://www.ibscertifications.org/certifications

EMSPro Specialty Certifications
https://emspro.org/specialist-fields-like-tactical-ems/

Similar Careers

Emergency Medical Manager

Medical Assistant

Physician Assistant

Registered Nurse

Firefighter

Police and Detective

CHAPTER 27

Pharmaceutical Sales Representative

Richard C Adrian, B.A

Education:	Bachelor's degree (Science/Business)	4 years
Income:	Entry-level $58,510 (range, $90,862 - $138,150)*	

Location will dictate initial salary. Technical/pharmaceutical representatives make higher salaries. Some metropolitan areas (e.g., Washington DC, NYC) have higher average entry level salaries. Representatives may also receive bonus-based sales. Additional benefits may include a company vehicle or car allowance, health insurance, 401k and stock options.

Why I Became a Pharmaceutical Sales Representative

Growing up, I always excelled at math and science. I was also super competitive and self-motivated. My parents raised me to know that success takes hard work. My father spent most of his career selling orthopedic implants, so my natural inclination was to follow him into sales. In college, I majored in Business Administration with a minor in Marketing. These choices allowed me to explore potential sales career options. During my senior year in college, I met a recruiter from Pfizer pharmaceuticals at a Career Fair. We discussed the healthcare industry and the need for quality salespeople. I realized that as the population ages, there is an increased demand for new and better medications. Sales representatives discuss new products with healthcare professionals so that they know how to use them appropriately to benefit patients. Unfortunately, I did not have a science background, so my sales career began with selling copiers and fax machines for Canon. The training I received from Canon taught me how to give specific sales presentations, but more importantly – it stressed the importance of gaining a commitment for a sale (also known as closing). After several successful years of working in sales at Canon, I had the opportunity to transition into a sales job with G.D. Searle. G.D. Searle was a small pharmaceutical company that marketed and sold medications mostly to primary care physician practices. After several years of sales success with G.D. Searle, I was promoted to one of their Hospital Sales Representatives.

As with any industry, there were numerous mergers and acquisitions, and I eventually started working for Pfizer Inc., the same company that sparked my initial interest in working in the healthcare field. Over the 20 plus years of working in the pharmaceutical industry, I have sold many products for many different diseases. I have been fortunate to develop some lasting relationships with clients who I now consider to be friends. The reason I continue to do what I do, and what satisfies me the most, is the impact my products have on the quality of patients' lives. There is nothing more satisfying and personally fulfilling than knowing that what you do impacts another human being's quality of life.

Overview

A pharmaceutical sales representative (Pharma Rep) is a person who has training in both business and clinical knowledge about a specific disease state, or different disease states. A Pharma Rep's goal is to increase awareness and use of his or her company's products. Pharma Reps travel within their assigned geography (or territory) to educate healthcare providers on the benefits and risks, costs and potential patient/practice implications for the company's products.

Specialties and Subspecialties

New Pharma Reps generally start by communicating with primary care or internal medicine physicians. Sometimes these doctors are general practitioners. The pharmaceutical company then may promote sales reps, based upon their sales performance, to call upon hospitals or health-systems or specialists, within their assigned territory. The assigned territory is the area or region where their practitioners are located. There are many different types of medical specialists. Some include pediatricians, geriatricians, endocrinologists, urologists or cardiologists, among others. Other clients may include Nurse Practitioners, Physician Assistants, Pharmacists, Nurses and Care Managers. The Health Insurance Portability and Accountability Act (HIPPA) guidelines strictly prevent Pharma Reps from directly interacting with patients.

After a sales representative has demonstrated success in sales along with gaining skills for promotion, other career paths could include Sales Management, Sales Training and Marketing. Pharmaceutical sales representatives should always actively interact with their manager (e.g., their boss) about their personal development to ensure they are moving their career in the proper direction and within company expectations.

A Pharma Rep's main goal is to achieve a sales quota or goal, market share growth (how much of the overall market your product is prescribed) and other business objectives, within an assigned territory. Successful pharmaceutical sales reps utilize consultative selling skills and in-depth clinical knowledge to drive sales results and impact customer support for their product(s). An example would be: discussing a clinical scenario with a physician and demonstrating how their company's product would be a better solution to manage their patient versus what he or she is currently doing. Reps must develop and implement strategic business plans which focus on growth (or increased use) of their product using business analytics, marketplace knowledge, competitor activity and clinical expertise. Marketplace knowledge is knowing your products as well as all competitor products, and how the medical profession currently is using them. This helps the Pharma Reps maximize time with their more important customers, as well as to have more impactful sales presentations.

Pharma Reps also need to identify and develop a network of key stakeholders who can impact their business at the local level, including healthcare providers, physician networks, local hospitals, pharmacies and large local employer groups (e.g., Google, Verizon, Coca-Cola, Hilton). Companies will require their reps to present marketing strategies and tactics in their assigned territory. The company will also provide a specific sales message when the FDA approves a new drug use (known as an indication) or when there is an insurance change for a product on their formulary. A formulary is a list of drug products available for use within a hospital or within a insurance plan. Not all drugs are included on the formulary. Pharma Reps work to include their drugs on formularies since this increases product use.

Requirements

There are a few different ways to pursue a career as a Pharma Rep. Most companies require at least a four-year bachelor's degree. Some universities offer a degree in pharmaceutical science, which include courses in chemistry, anatomy, biology, health science and business. Students who enroll in traditional science majors can add a minor in business to enhance their qualifications. Pursuing a degree in business is another way to become a pharmaceutical sales representative. However, you may need to begin your career as a traditional sales representative (not a pharmaceutical representative) and transition later into the pharmaceutical field. Examples of traditional sales careers would be for office equipment (companies like Xerox or Canon), insurance companies or in financial product sales. These traditional sales jobs provide individuals with training focused on delivering formal product presentations to different group sizes. A minimum of two to three years of successful sales experience is sometimes preferred, in lieu of a science focused degree, prior to transitioning into a job in pharmaceutical sales.

Pharmaceutical companies have both initial and ongoing training that is mandatory for all their employed representatives to complete. Some of this training includes both compliance and professional conduct. This training is focused on the rules and regulations of the U.S. FDA. This training ensures that Pharma Reps interact with healthcare providers in a lawful and satisfactory manner. The Pharmaceutical Research and Manufacturers Association (PhRMA), also known as "Pharma," has established guidelines for Pharma Reps, to use during their interactions with healthcare professionals. This is known as the "PharmaCode." All Pharmaceutical sales representatives must follow the PharmaCode. By not adhering to these guidelines, Pharma Reps are subject to discipline by both their employer and the FDA. This discipline may include job termination, significant fines and jail time. The Sunshine Act, a provision of the Affordable Care Act (2010), is one example of increased transparency by which reporting of all payments and gifts to a specific healthcare provider is mandatory. This law requires documentation of all attendees at sponsored lunches and speaker dinners to accurately reflect the monetary value of services provided. Inaccurate reporting could result in fines for the company and disciplinary action for the representative.

There are several personality traits that make for successful Pharma Reps. They have strong communication skills (both oral and written) which are critical for discussing complex clinical data with both healthcare providers and internal colleagues. Reps must be self-motivated, managing most of their daily activities. Reps must have drive, ambition and individual accountability, characteristics present in top performers. Organizational and critical thinking skills enable reps to develop strategic business plans for their assigned territory to increase sales results. An outgoing personality helps representatives to meet new customers, develop relationships and expand their customer base. There are several resources available to assess and develop these traits. Strength Finders 2.0 gives the individual an assessment and summarizes his or her five core strengths. Strength Finders 2.0 can help decide which job in the healthcare industry best suits their core strengths.

A Day in the Life of a Pharmaceutical Sales Representative

My work week usually begins on a Sunday night where I review my strategic business plan for the week. I look at which physicians have office hours in the territory where I plan to be that week. As a specialty representative, my day starts at the hospital, going to different units where they use my product. Once there, I would discuss patient cases who may be appropriate candidates for my product. Several healthcare professionals in a hospital may be involved in selecting a drug. These individuals might include: 1) the attending physician who would order and start the product; 2) the clinical pharmacist who would ensure there are no drug/drug interactions, and that the proper dose of the medication is correct, and that the patient is appropriately monitored for effectiveness and adverse effects of the drug; and 3) the social worker/care or case manager who would ensure a smooth transition for the patient, from the hospital to home, and whether his or her insurance covers the medication once the patient is no longer in the hospital. When I finish at the hospital, I go to the offices of my key targeted clients (e.g., prescribers). Another part of my day, besides client interactions, revolves around long-term projects to expand opportunities to encourage medical professionals to use my product on a more widespread basis. Examples of this would include: 1) obtaining formulary access for my product; 2) impacting hospital guidelines to use my product, also known as protocols/pathways; and/or 3) connecting local experts with high level people in my company to discuss potential opportunities for research and other collaborative projects.

My description above would be the typical day for a Pharm Rep covering a major metropolitan area or an urban territory. For a rep in a rural area, the territory is usually much larger in size, sometimes covering an entire state or multiple states. For these Pharma Reps, it is imperative to develop a strategic map of their territory to ensure that they see all their key customers with the right frequency, to maximize their business. In the Pharma world, this is known as routing. These Pharma Reps may have substantial amounts of driving or flying as part of their day, as well as the potential for overnight stays in their territory.

In a recent survey of Medical/Pharma Reps, 76% of respondents said they are somewhat or very satisfied in their jobs. The reps' comments regarding their satisfaction included: the ability to make a difference; the quality of their products; competitive compensation; promotion structure; and mentorship and coaching opportunities.

Search and Explore

The National Association of Pharmaceutical Sales Representatives
http://www.napsronline.org/

News releases and job center
http://www.cafepharma.com

The Pharmaceutical Research and Manufacturers Association
http://www.phrma.org

Strengths Finder
http://strengths.gallup.com/110440/About-StrengthsFinder-20.aspx

Pharmaceutical Industry Updates
http://www.pharmexec.com

Similar Careers

Specialty Pharmaceutical Sales Representatives (high-cost oral, inhaled or injectable medications used to treat complex conditions)

Diagnostic Imaging Sales Representatives (X-Ray, magnetic resonance imaging, computed tomography [CT] machines)

Medical Device Sales Representatives (thermometers, gloves, bedpans)

Health Informational Technology (IT)/Software Sales Representatives (health/hospital system electronic platforms)

Capital Equipment/Durable Medical Equipment Sales Representatives (braces, wheelchairs, oxygen tanks, nebulizers, hospital beds)

Surgical Device Sales Representatives (prosthetic joints, pacemakers)

Biotechnology Sales Representatives (biological products, cancer immunotherapies)

CHAPTER 28

Medical Writer

Michele B Kaufman, PharmD., BCGP

Education:	Bachelor's degree	4 years
Optional:	Master of Science (Biomedical Writing)	1 - 2 years
	Doctor of Pharmacy	4 years
	Doctor of Philosophy	4 years
Median income:	$70,000*	

*Fulltime medical writer. Medical writers can also be paid by the job or by the number of words in the assignment

Why I Became a Medical Writer

I became a pharmacist first and then started my own medical writing company. As to how I became a pharmacist...I always knew I would attend college. That is how it was in my family. My parents met as undergraduate students at Brooklyn College in New York, married and then moved to Pittsburgh together for graduate school. My Dad pursued his Doctor of Philosophy degree in Organic Chemistry and my Mom obtained her Master's degree in Education.

As a child, I always had more of an inclination towards science. I had my chemistry set and loved performing experiments. When I ran out of chemicals, my Dad would always help. He would come into school and give cool science demonstrations to my classes, like how to make silk. I had the chance to do some neat science projects throughout the years. I thought I would pursue a career as a chemist, as my Dad did. I enjoyed chemistry but was also interested in toxicology and how drugs work in the human body. Also, the thought of going to school for ten years before I could really "work" as a chemist was pretty daunting to a 16 or 17 year old. Having lived through most of the 1960s and all of the 1970s, there was considerable anti-drug (and drug) education. I remember commercials on television about psychedelic drugs, and I always wondered "How do those work? Why are they so bad? What are they doing to the brain?" I wanted to understand the pharmacology of these reactions. I was also trying to figure out how to meld my interests into a career. I also thought about having a career in music since I play the saxophone. I hadn't thought about pharmacy until I started looking into colleges. While perusing some college catalogues and visiting colleges, I looked for both chemistry, medicinal chemistry and pharmacy. I decided I would continue playing music as a hobby, because succeeding as a career musician is very difficult. I applied to a small number of colleges and universities and would decide on my "major" following "acceptances." I was accepted to all the schools where I had applied. I had a decision to make. I visited the University of Rhode Island (URI) in Kingston and was so impressed by the College of Pharmacy, the campus and all the faculty and students who I met that I decided to enroll and pursue a Bachelor of Science degree in Pharmacy. It was the best choice I made. I love being a pharmacist. I have worked in many different aspects, and I have learned from them all. Like my co-author, I landed my first independent retail pharmacy job by going store to store with my resume, until someone would hire me. I lived in New Jersey, in Rutgers College of Pharmacy territory, and it was incredibly difficult to find a job, since I was away at school and those students were all "local." Obtaining my first job in a pharmacy was great experience, and the two pharmacist owners kept me in the pharmacy area filling prescriptions, I did not stock greeting cards or run the lottery machine. I was a "professional" and they valued me, as I valued learning from them. Subsequently, my mom made a connection for me through a career fair at her school, and I obtained a job as a pharmacy intern/student at a local medical center during the next summer. I learned new and interesting skills as a hospital pharmacy employee that still apply to what I do today as a hospital pharmacist. When I earned my BS in Pharmacy, I also received a minor in Music. I play the saxophone in community bands in New York City. My love of music led me to meeting my spouse in a New York City Community Band in early 2001.

I always enjoyed researching information to find answers. While I was in training for my PharmD, one of our mandatory clinical rotations was in a hospital-based drug information center. Although I had a broken hand at the time, I still enjoyed researching information for healthcare providers to use in improving patient care. In addition, I was lucky to have a very skilled and knowledgeable research mentor who worked with me on improving my writing and editing skills. As "drug experts," one of our major responsibilities as pharmacists is to provide drug information. We answer simple and complex patient-specific (or non-patient specific) drug related questions. Realizing how much I really enjoyed doing this, I had the opportunity to participate in a drug information rotation in the Medical Affairs Department at Upjohn Pharmaceuticals in Kalamazoo, MI.

While on this rotation, I was involved in writing answers to medication specific questions about Upjohn's pharmaceutical products. These questions were from healthcare providers all over the globe. It was here that I refined my medical writing skills as scientists (mostly pharmacists) critiqued my writing and editing. Following this rotation, I realized that I wanted to continue to research and write, while also continuing to work as a clinician.

Therefore, in choosing my "next step," I looked for a job or post-graduate program (residency or fellowship) where I could round with the medical team to improve patient care, and improve my drug information skills, and have the opportunity to publish. This led me to pursue a one-year Drug Information Fellowship at the URI Drug Information Center at Roger Williams Medical Center in Providence. During my fellowship, I had the opportunity to be involved in a state-run adverse drug reaction monitoring program, which is where I developed my interest in pharmacovigilance (or drug safety; see glossary). In addition to my work in pharmacovigilance, I also was able to round with the medical and cardiac care unit teams, teach, write and conduct research. I published numerous peer-reviewed articles during this year, as well as many other articles, including newsletter articles. In the subsequent year, I pursued a faculty position at St. John's University College of Pharmacy in Jamaica, NY. In a tenure track position, the moniker was "publish or perish," so I continued to publish, participate in research and teach. I also joined the state health-system pharmacy society, the New York State Council of Health-system Pharmacists (NYSCHP), and the local chapter. I became a Contributing Editor of the *NYSCHP Pharmacy Journal*, a position I held for over 10 years.

When I left academia, I took a position in the corporate office of a managed care company in NYC. Here I was involved in formulary management activities, writing for internal and external healthcare professional audiences in newsletters, and internal documents for medication approvals, acting as a drug information resource for the health plan's hundreds of healthcare providers, providing clinical support to patients and healthcare providers, trending drugs in the approval pipeline to help determine when they would become available for use, providing case management programs for Medicare/geriatric patients and committee work. While working at the health plan, particularly as it related to drug trending and geriatric case management, I started to pick up freelance writing projects. I became acquainted with the medical education company, Prime® Inc., who provided CE/CME to case managers and other healthcare professionals. I became a pharmacy consultant, and content peer reviewer for Prime® Inc., as well as an editor for their "pharmacist specific website." After I left my position at the health plan, I started a part-time (remote; working off-site) position with them as a Senior Medical Writer. While working for Prime® Inc, I started my own medical writing company, PRN Communications, Inc. It was around this time that I joined the American Medical Writers Association (AMWA) and started attending local meetings in NYC where I had the opportunity to meet other medical writers, and network for other freelance writing jobs. In addition, through some other professional connections, I was able to pick up steady freelance writing work for four different print publications, and other jobs on an "as needed" basis. I continued writing full-time for almost two years, when I decided to reconnect with clinical pharmacy and direct patient care and connect with one of the local pharmacy colleges to do some teaching. I first met Mary Choy while attending a pharmacy meeting. She was in academia and started a medical writing elective at the college. She invited me to speak to her students about a career as a medical writer. We also started collaborating on writing projects and involving students in writing and presenting research at regional and national meetings. While I was still managing my company, a pharmacy director hired me to round with the medical teams and provide direct patient care, act as a drug information resource, provide formulary activities and manage the adverse drug reaction monitoring and reporting (e.g. pharmacovigilance) services. Eventually, I decided to return to hospital pharmacy full-time and continue medical writing on a freelance basis. Currently, I am a writer for two drug information columns in two different publications. I also have a Pharmacovigilance column in *P&T Journal* and I still consult for

Prime® Inc. I really love writing and editing. My involvement in direct patient care helps me keep up-to-date with current medications, drug safety issues and prescribing trends, which in turn gives me new writing ideas.

Overview

Most medical writers enter the field without formal training. Like me and many others who I know, we started out with a pharmacy, medical or scientific degree. We worked (or work) in those fields as scientists, physicians or pharmacists, before transitioning into medical writing as a full-time occupation or in a freelance capacity. Other individuals have entered the medical writing field from a non-science background. These individuals include journalists, who developed into medical writers as a career through health and medicine article writing, or English or Communications majors. Some medical writers have a master's degree in Public Health. Many technical writers, of which medical writing is a subcategory, earn a bachelor's degree in English or journalism and/ or a specific field. Medical writers do not need to be PhD trained to find work. If you like to write, you can become involved in STEM in elementary school or later. You can also join science groups and offer to write about these in a school or local newsletter, website or blog. Perhaps there are other science/ medical-based websites where you can try your hand at writing. Take writing and science classes, and always look for an opportunity to write.

Some colleges offer certificates in writing and editing such as in marketing writing and regulatory writing; medical writing and editing; or even a biomedical writing master's degree. The Certificate in Marketing Writing focuses on publications. A certificate in regulatory writing focuses on preparing documents for initial and continuing approval of therapies at the U.S. FDA. One certificate in medical writing and editing ensures students are trained in the industry standard American Medical Association (AMA) Style Manual. Coursework can include accessing medical research, using appropriate terminology and designing and presenting visual data. Students learn the fundamentals of medical writing and editing and discuss best practices and related medical research. One of the certificate courses has no required prerequisite classes, and students can take the coursework that works best for them, as a four course or six course (advanced) certificate.

Some of these more advanced certificates are for practicing professionals who want to further their careers or gain additional training and credentialing in the biomedical writing field.

At least two professional organizations offer certifications. The Board of Editors in Life Sciences is a professional organization that evaluates the proficiency of manuscript editors in the life sciences and awards editing credentials based on passing a proficiency exam. The AMWA, in collaboration with the Medical Writing Certification Commission (MWCC), has developed the Medical Writer Certified (MWC°) credential that defines the scope of medical writing practice and distinguishes individuals in the field through exam-based professional certification. These courses and certifications are optional.

Specialties and Subspecialties

Medical writers prepare different types of scientific documents which include regulatory and research-related documents, disease or drug-related educational and promotional literature, journal abstracts and manuscripts for publication, healthcare website content, professional newsletters (e.g., *Physician's Letter*, *Pharmacist's Letter*, *The Medical Letter*) and websites (e.g., MedPage Today, Medscape), health-related magazines or health-related news articles, brochures, blogs, among other types of information. One can also write for healthcare organizations or government agencies (e.g., FDA, National Institutes of Health, Centers for Disease Control, State/Local Health Department), consulting firms, nonprofit organizations, or professional societies, to name a few.

Health writing is medical writing which includes information such as educational material and other content that is directed towards consumers or patients. *Scientific writing* involves mostly academic publications, science journalism and other forms of technical writing.

Medical writing subspecialties include:

- **Regulatory writing** is almost always completed by clinicians or scientists who communicate information to government agencies, heads of compliance departments and other reviewers. This is usually in relation to summarizing data from clinical trials in support of submitting data for drug, device or vaccine/biologic approval. This is usually for a pharmaceutical, device or a vaccine/biologic company.

- **Promotional writing** is educational material for a specific product "brand." Basically, it is regulated marketing for the healthcare industry, for pharmaceutical promotion. A promotional writer can work for a pharmaceutical or other "brand/product" company, or for an advertising or other "marketing" type of agency. Promotional writing may also include sales training, drug monographs, advertising copy or planning of publications.

- **Medical education or CME** is for healthcare providers to maintain their license to practice. CME provides programming, board-review products, disease monographs and other educational materials to keep practitioners educated and current in their respective fields. CME educates readers without bias for or against any specific brand or product.

Requirements

Obtaining a bachelor's degree is key to writing. If you do not have a scientific degree, obtaining a certificate in some aspect of medical writing/editing improves your prospects of obtaining work as a medical writer and/or editor. The Overview section explains some of the available courses.

A Day in The Life of a Medical Writer

While I managed my own medical writing company, I was always on the lookout for interesting topics for my articles. I subscribe to several different online resources in abstracts and news articles that provide drug-related information. In addition, I receive "daily briefings" from many professional organizations that also provide drug/disease information. Each day I review the information in these sources for potential topics related to the columns that I write. For instance, I write the Drug Update column for *The Rheumatologist*, so I research new information on rheumatology-related drugs and drug safety. I also look at information related to co-morbidities (other conditions/diseases that these patients may have) in this population of rheumatology patients. I usually write about new data on drugs that I obtain from performing a literature search from the National Library of Medicine journal database (a more detailed and formalized information retrieval process), professional society websites, disease-state diagnosis and management guidelines and the web. I choose different types of information for this readership, which is mostly U.S. based rheumatology practitioners, but some international practitioners. These practitioners include physicians (rheumatologists and internists), nurse practitioners, physician assistants, nurses, pharmacists, orthopedic surgeons and other healthcare professionals who practice, research or teach in the field of rheumatology. After I complete a project, I invoice (or bill) the Editor of the respective publication for the work completed. I budget my time to complete my projects in advance of the deadline, or at the deadline. I also attend professional meetings and CE programs to network and obtain new writing ideas. I also travel to national conferences to write about recent advances and new clinical cases.

Search and Explore

American Society of Health-Systems Pharmacy
http://www.ashp.org

American Medical Writers Association
http://www.amwa.org (Essential skills in medical writing)

Science Writers in New York
http://www.swiny.org

University of the Sciences
https://www.usciences.edu/misher-college-of-arts-and-sciences/biomedical-writing-ms-certificates/

University of Chicago Graham School Medical Writing and Editing Certificate
https://grahamschool.uchicago.edu/medical-writing-and-editing-certificate

Board of Editors in the Life Sciences
http://www.bels.org

Hitt Medical Writing
http://www.hittmedicalwriting.com/thehittlist.html

Similar Careers

Medical Scribe - BS in medical field, pre-health/pre-PA students and certificate

References

Surgical Technologist (Chapter 1)

Bureau of Labor Statistics, U.S. Department of Labor, Occupational Outlook Handbook: Surgical Technologists. https://www.bls.gov/ooh/healthcare/surgical-technologists.htm September 2019

US News and World Report Best Jobs Surgical Technologist Published January 18, 2019 http://money.usnews.com/careers/best-jobs/surgical-technologist

Fried JP. Trading Up to Careers in the Operating Room Published December 10, 2006. http://www.nytimes.com/2006/12/10/jobs/10homefront.html

US News and World Report Best Jobs Published January 8, 2019 https://money.usnews.com/careers/best-jobs/surgical-technologist

Pharmacist (Chapter 2)

Bureau of Labor Statistics, U.S. Department of Labor, Occupational Outlook Handbook: Pharmacists. https://www.bls.gov/ooh/healthcare/pharmacists.htm September 2019

Academic Pharmacy's Vital Statistics. American Association of Colleges of Pharmacy. Published 2019 https://www.aacp.org/article/academic-pharmacys-vital-statistics.

US News and World Report Best Jobs. Published January 8, 2018 https://money.usnews.com/careers/best-jobs/pharmacist.

US News and World Report. How to Become a Pharmacist. Published July 22, 2019. https://www.usnews.com/education/best-graduate-schools/articles/2019-07-22/

how-to-get-into-pharmacy-school-and-become-a-pharmacist

American College of Clinical Pharmacy (ACCP) http://www.accp.com

Board of Pharmacy Specialties (BPS) http://www.bpsweb.org

American Pharmacists Association (APhA) http://www.apha.org

American Society of Health-System Pharmacists (ASHP) https://www.ashp.org/

Pharmacy Technician (Chapter 3)

Bureau of Labor Statistics, U.S. Department of Labor, Occupational Outlook Handbook: Pharmacy Technicians. https://www.bls.gov/ooh/healthcare/pharmacy-technicians.htm September 2019

Pharmacy Technician Certification Board (PTCB) Certified Pharmacy Technician (CPhT) Map and Regulatory Snapshot, Published December 31, 2017 http://www.ptcb.org/who-we-serve/pharmacy-technicians/cphts-state-regulatory-map#.WPZVPPnyvRY

Bright D, Adams AJ. Pharmacy technician–administered vaccines in Idaho. *Am J Health-Syst Pharm* 2017;74:2033-2034.

McKeirnan KC, Frazier KR, Nguyen M, MacLean LG. Training pharmacy technicians to administer immunizations. *J Am Pharm Assoc* 2018;58:174-178.

Burke R. Update from PTCB from the NYSCHP News Brief. Published March/April 2019;6:7-9. https://nyschp.memberclicks.net/assets/docs/Newsletters/April%20Newsbrief%20NYSCHP.pdf

U.S. News and World Report Best Jobs 2019 Published January 8, 2019 https://money.usnews.com/careers/best-jobs/pharmacy-technician

Osteopathic Physician (Chapter 4)

Bureau of Labor Statistics, U.S. Department of Labor, Occupational Outlook Handbook, Physicians and Surgeons. https://www.bls.gov/ooh/healthcare/physicians-and-surgeons.htm September 2019

Doctors of Osteopathic Medicine Published 2019 http://doctorsthatdo.org/

Doctors of Osteopathic Medicine - the DO difference Published 2019 http://doctorsthatdo.org/difference

Doctors of Osteopathic Medicine - Osteopathic Manipulative Treatment Published 2019 http://doctorsthatdo.org/difference/osteopathic-manipulative-treatment

American Academy of Osteopathy - Osteopathic Medical Education Published 2019 https://www.academyofosteopathy.org/osteopathic-medical-education

DiGiovanna E, Schiowitz S, Dowling D. An Osteopathic Approach to Diagnosis and Treatment, 2nd ed. Philadelphia: Lippincott Raven 1997

Akademia Osteopatii http://akademiaosteopatii.pl/osteopatia/andrew-taylor-still/?lang=en

American Association of Medical Colleges Careers in Medicine Specialty list Published 2019 https://www.aamc.org/cim/specialty/exploreoptions/list/

Accreditation Council for Graduate Medical Education Published 2019 http://www.acgme.org/What-We-Do/Recognition/Osteopathic-Recognition US News and World Report Best Jobs 2019 Published January 8, 2019 https://money.usnews.com/careers/best-jobs/physician

Registered Nurse (Chapter 5)

Bureau of Labor Statistics, U.S. Department of Labor, Occupational Outlook Handbook: Registered Nurses. https://www.bls.gov/ooh/healthcare/registered-nurses.htm September 2019

Bureau of Labor Statistics, U.S. Department of Labor, Occupational Outlook Handbook: Licensed Practical and Licensed Vocational Nurses https://www.bls.gov/ooh/healthcare/licensed-practical-and-licensed-vocational-nurses.htm September 2019

National Council of State Boards of Nursing, Inc. Quarterly Examination Statistics for 2019. Published 2019 https://www.ncsbn.org/NCLEX_Stats_2019.pdf

Complete List of Common Nursing Certifications Published July 8, 2017 https://nurse.org/articles/nursing-certifications-credentials-list/

US News and World Report Best Jobs 2019 Published January 8, 2019 https://money.usnews.com/careers/best-jobs/registered-nurse

US News and Word Report Best Jobs 2019 Published January 8, 2019 https://money.usnews.com/careers/best-jobs/nurse-practitioner

US News and Word Report Best Jobs 2019 Published January 8, 2019 https://money.usnews.com/careers/best-jobs/nurse-midwife

Certified Registered Nurse Anesthetist (Chapter 6)

Bureau of Labor Statistics, U.S. Department of Labor, Occupational Outlook Handbook: Nurse Anesthetists, Nurse Midwives, and Nurse Practitioners. https://

www.bls.gov/ooh/healthcare/nurse-anesthetists-nurse-midwives-and-nurse-practitioners.htm September 2019

American Association of Nurse Anesthetists Certified Registered Nurse Anesthetists Fact Sheet Published February 28, 2019 https://www.aana.com/membership/become-a-crna/crna-fact-sheet

American Association of Nurse Anesthetists Published 2018 *Standards for Nurse Anesthesia Practice*. https://www.aana.com/docs/default-source/practice-aana-com-web-documents-(all)/standards-for-nurse-anesthesia-practice.pdf?sfvrsn=e00049b1_2

Council on Accreditation of Nurse Anesthesia Educational Programs http://home.coa.us.com/accredited-programs/Pages/CRNA-School-Search.aspx

American Association of Nurse Anesthetists Advanced Pain Management Fellowship Program https://www.aana.com/ce-education/pain-management/advanced-pain-management-fellowship-program

US News and World Best Jobs 2019 Report Published April 15, 2019 https://money.usnews.com/careers/best-jobs/nurse-anesthetist

Managed Care Case Manager (Chapter 7)

Salary.com Case Management Salaries Published March 28, 2019 https://www1.salary.com/case-manager-salaries.html

Leonard M, Miller E. *Nursing Case Management and Resource Manual,* 4th ed. Maryland: The American Nursing Association, 2015.

Commission for Case Management Certification, Case Management Certification Published 2018 https://ccmcertification.org/get-certified/certification/ccmr-eligibility-glance

Physician Assistant (Chapter 8)

Bureau of Labor Statistics, U.S. Department of Labor, Occupational Outlook Handbook: Physician Assistants. https://www.bls.gov/ooh/healthcare/physician-assistants.htm September 2019

US News and World Report Best Jobs, Published January 8, 2019 http://money.usnews.com/careers/best-jobs/physician-assistant

Accreditation Review Commission on Education for the Physician Assistant, Inc. Published 2019 http://www.arc-pa.org/accreditation/accredited-programs/

National Commission on Certification of Physician Assistants Published 2019 https://www.nccpa.net/earn-speciality-certificates

Banks E. NCCPA Specialty Certificate Program Adds Certified PAs to Its Roll Press Release http://prodcmsstoragesa.blob.core.windows.net/uploads/files/PressReleaseCAQRecipients2018.pdf

Veterinarian (Chapter 9)

Bureau of Labor Statistics, U.S. Department of Labor, Occupational Outlook Handbook: Veterinarians. https://www.bls.gov/ooh/healthcare/veterinarians.htm September 2019

US News and World Report Best Healthcare Jobs Published January 9, 2019 https://money.usnews.com/careers/best-jobs/veterinarian

Phlebotomist (Chapter 10)

Bureau of Labor Statistics, U.S. Department of Labor, Occupational Outlook Handbook: Phlebotomists. https://www.bls.gov/ooh/healthcare/phlebotomists.htm September 2019

Discover Information About Health Care & Medical Science Careers! Published 2019 https://chrms.org/information-about-obtaining-a-phlebotomy-certification/

Phlebotomy Career Guide and Outlook, Published 2013 http://www.phlebotomyguide.org/

US News and World Report Best Health Care Jobs Published January 8, 2019 https://money.usnews.com/careers/best-jobs/phlebotomist

Bureau of Labor Statistics Occupational Outlook Handbook Phlebotomists Published April 12, 2019 https://www.bls.gov/ooh/healthcare/phlebotomists.htm#tab-8

Dentist (Chapter 11)

Bureau of Labor Statistics, U.S. Department of Labor, Occupational Outlook Handbook: Dentists. https://www.bls.gov/ooh/healthcare/dentists.htm September 2019

Jumpstart Your Dental Career in High School American Dental Education Association Published October 6, 2015 https://www.youtube.com/watch?v=bXMAQzViq-8

The American Dental Education Association http://www.adea.org/GoDental/Application_Prep/The_Admissions_Process/DAT_(Dental_Admission_Test).aspx

American Dental Association http://www.ada.org/

American Dental Education Association Published 2019 http://www.adea.org/dentalfellow/

US News and World Report Best Healthcare Jobs Published January 8, 2019 http://money.usnews.com/careers/best-jobs/dentist

Dental Hygienist (Chapter 12)

Bureau of Labor Statistics, U.S. Department of Labor, Occupational Outlook Handbook: Dental Hygienists. https://www.bls.gov/ooh/healthcare/dental-hygienists.htm September 2019

US News and World Report Best Jobs Published January 10, 2019 https://money.usnews.com/careers/best-jobs/dental-hygienist

Dietitian Nutritionist (Chapter 13)

Bureau of Labor Statistics, U.S. Department of Labor, Occupational Outlook Handbook: Dietitians and Nutritionists. https://www.bls.gov/ooh/healthcare/dietitians-and-nutritionists.htm September 2019

What is a Registered Dietitian Nutritionist? Published 2019 http://www.eatrightpro.org/resources/about-us/what-is-an-rdn-and-dtr/what-is-a-registered-dietitian-nutritionist

Commission on Dietetic Registration. Published 2019 https://www.cdrnet.org.

US News and World Report Best Jobs Published January 9, 2019 https://money.usnews.com/careers/best-jobs/dietitian-and-nutritionist

Orthodontist (Chapter 14)

Bureau of Labor Statistics, U.S. Department of Labor, Occupational Employment Statistics: Orthodontists. https://www.bls.gov/oes/2017/may/oes291023.htm March 2018

US News and World Report Best Jobs Published January 8, 2019 https://money.usnews.com/careers/best-jobs/orthodontist

Podiatrist (Chapter 15)

Bureau of Labor Statistics, U.S. Department of Labor, Occupational Outlook Handbook: Podiatrists. https://www.bls.gov/ooh/healthcare/podiatrists.htm September 2019

2014 Podiatric Practice Survey, Discovering Podiatric Medicine Chapter 1 Published 2014 http://www.aacpm.org/wp-content/uploads/2017-Income-Page.pdf

The Council on Podiatric Medical Education Published May 2019 https://www.cpme.org/colleges/content.cfm?ItemNumber=2425

US News and World Report Best Jobs Published January 8, 2019 https://money.usnews.com/careers/best-jobs/podiatrist

Biomedical Engineer (Chapter 16)

Bureau of Labor Statistics, U.S. Department of Labor, Occupational Outlook Handbook: Biomedical Engineers. https://www.bls.gov/ooh/architecture-and-engineering/biomedical-engineers.htm September 2019

Goudreau J. The 15 Most Valuable College Majors. Published May 15, 2012 https://www.forbes.com/sites/jennagoudreau/2012/05/15/best-top-most-valuable-college-majors-degrees/#1441ad94dcc4

US News and World Report Best Jobs Published January 10, 2018 https://money.usnews.com/careers/best-jobs/biomedical-engineer

Clinical/Counseling Psychologist (Chapter 17)

Bureau of Labor Statistics, U.S. Department of Labor, Occupational Outlook Handbook: Psychologists. https://www.bls.gov/ooh/Life-Physical-and-Social-Science/Psychologists.htm September 2019.

Lin L, Christidis P, Stamm K. 2015 Salaries in Psychology Published May 2017 https://www.apa.org/workforce/publications/2015-salaries/index

American Psychological Association Divisions by Number Published in 2019 http://www.apa.org/about/division/index.aspx Last Accessed May 15, 2019

American Psychological Association Divisions by Topic Published in 2019 http://www.apa.org/about/division/index.aspx?tab=2

US News & World Report Top 100 Jobs. Published January 8, 2019 https://money.usnews.com/careers/best-jobs/psychologist

US News & World Report Top 100 Jobs. Published January 8, 2019 https://money.usnews.com/careers/best-jobs/school-psychologist

Physical Therapist (Chapter 18)

Bureau of Labor Statistics, U.S. Department of Labor, Occupational Outlook

Handbook: Physical Therapists. https://www.bls.gov/ooh/healthcare/physical-therapists.htm September 2019

Physical Therapist Centralized Application Service Prerequisites 2017-2018 Published January 4, 2017 http://www.ptcas.org/uploadedFiles/PTCASorg/Directory/Prerequisites/PTCASCoursePreReqsSummary.pdf

Physical Therapist Centralized Application Service list of non-PTCAS institutions programs Published January 2019 http://www.ptcas.org/ptcas/public/allprograms.aspx?listorder=nonptcas&navID=10737426794

American Physical Therapy Association. Who Are Physical Therapists? Published March 11, 2019 http://www.apta.org/AboutPTs/

The Federation of State Boards of Physical Therapy Published 2019 http://www.fsbpt.org/ExamCandidates.aspx

American Board of Physical Therapy Residency and Fellowship Education Published 2019 http://www.abpts.org/Certification/About/

American Board of Physical Therapy Residency and Fellowship Education Published 2019 http://www.abptrfe.org/Home.aspx

American Physical Therapy Association. Who Are Physical Therapist Assistants? Published on March 11, 2019 http://www.apta.org/AboutPTAs/ Last Accessed

US News and World Report Best Jobs Published January 8, 2019 https://money.usnews.com/careers/best-jobs/physical-therapist

Occupational Therapist (Chapter 19)

Bureau of Labor Statistics, U.S. Department of Labor, Occupational Outlook Handbook: Occupational Therapists. https://www.bls.gov/ooh/healthcare/occupational-therapists.htm September 2019

US News and World Report Best Jobs 2019 Occupational Therapist Overview Published January 8, 2019 http://money.usnews.com/careers/best-jobs/occupational-therapist

Social Worker (Chapter 20)

Bureau of Labor Statistics, U.S. Department of Labor, Occupational Outlook Handbook: Social Workers. https://www.bls.gov/ooh/community-and-social-service/social-workers.htm September 2019

US News and World Report http://money.usnews.com/careers/best-jobs/clinical-social-worker Published January 10, 2018

Bureau of Labor Statistics Occupational Outlook Handbook Psychologists Published April 12, 2019 https://www.bls.gov/ooh/life-physical-and-social-science/psychologists.htm#tab-8

Music Therapist/Mental Health Counselor (Chapter 21)

What is the potential salary of a music therapist? https://www.musictherapy.org/faq/#337

Music Therapy Association Inc. 2016 AMTA Member Survey & Workforce Analysis: A Descriptive, Statistical Profile of the AMTA Membership and Music Therapy Community. 2016:12.

NYU Steinhardt: Nordoff-Robbins Center for Music Therapy. Nordoff-Robbins Music Therapy. http://steinhardt.nyu.edu/music/nordoff/therapy/nordoff

The Academy of Neurologic Music Therapy. International Training Institutes in NMT. https://nmtacademy.co/training-opportunities/nmt-training-institute/

About Guided Imagery and Music: The Bonny Method of Guided Imagery and Music (GIM). http://www.gim-trainings.com/about.html

Diane Austin. Music Psychotherapy http://dianeaustin.com/music/

Priestley, M. (1994). *Essays on Analytical Music Therapy*. Phoenixville, PA: Barcelona Publishers.

Malchiodi C. Creative Arts Therapy and Expressive Arts Therapy Published June 30, 2014 https://www.psychologytoday.com/blog/arts-and-health/201406/creative-arts-therapy-and-expressive-arts-therapy

American Music Therapy Association: What is Music Therapy. http://www.musictherapy.org/about/musictherapy/

The Certification Board for Music Therapists. http://www.cbmt.org/

NYU Steinhardt: Nordoff-Robbins Center for Music Therapy. Audition/Interview Information. http://steinhardt.nyu.edu/music/nordoff/training/audition/

Music Therapy Can Comfort and Soothe Premature Infants and Parents Published April 15, 2013 https://www.aap.org/en-us/about-the-aap/aap-press-room/Pages/Music-Therapy-Can-Comfort-and-Soothe-Premature-Infants-and-Parents.aspx

Art Therapist/Mental Health Counselor (Chapter 22)

Bureau of Labor Statistics Occupational Employment and Wages, Published April 2015 https://www.bls.gov/careeroutlook/2015/youre-a-what/art-therapist.htm

Torpey E. Your a What? Art Therapist. Published April 2015 https://www.bls.gov/careeroutlook/2015/youre-a-what/art-therapist.htm

Occupational Outlook Handbook Recreational Therapists Published September 2019 https://www.bls.gov/ooh/healthcare/recreational-therapists.htm

Medical Imaging Technologist (Chapter 23)

Bureau of Labor Statistics (BLS). Radiologic and MRI Technologists. Published September 2019. *Occupational Outlook Handbook*. https://www.bls.gov/ooh/healthcare/radiologic-technologists.htm

Bureau of Labor Statistics (BLS). Nuclear Medicine Technologists. Published September 2019. *Occupational Outlook Handbook*. http://www.bls.gov/ooh/healthcare/nuclear-medicine-technologists.htm

Bureau of Labor Statistics (BLS). Radiation Therapists. *Occupational Outlook Handbook*. Published September 2019. https://www.bls.gov/ooh/healthcare/radiation-therapists.htm

US News and World Report Best Health Care Jobs Published January 9, 2019 http://money.usnews.com/careers/best-jobs/radiologic-technologist

US News and World Report Best Health Care Support Jobs Published January 9, 2019 https://money.usnews.com/careers/best-jobs/diagnostic-medical-sonographer

US News and World Report Best Health Care Support Jobs Published January 9, 2019 https://money.usnews.com/careers/best-jobs/mri-technologist

Clinical Laboratory Technologist (Chapter 24)

Bureau of Labor Statistics, U.S. Department of Labor, Occupational Outlook Handbook, 2018 Edition, Medical and Clinical Laboratory Technologists and Technicians Published September 2019 https://www.bls.gov/ooh/healthcare/medical-and-clinical-laboratory-technologists-and-technicians.htm

New York City Public Health Laboratory, New York City Department of Health website Published 2019 https://www1.nyc.gov/site/doh/providers/reporting-and-services/public-health-lab.page

U.S. News & World Report Best Health Care Support Jobs. Published January 10, 2019 https://money.usnews.com/careers/best-jobs/clinical-laboratory-technician

Speech and Language Pathologist (Chapter 25)

Bureau of Labor Statistics, U.S. Department of Labor, Occupational Outlook Handbook: Speech-Language Pathologists. https://www.bls.gov/ooh/healthcare/speech-language-pathologists.htm September 2019

US News and World Report Best Healthcare Jobs Published January 8, 2019 https://money.usnews.com/careers/best-jobs/speech-language-pathologist

American Speech-Language-Hearing Association https://www.asha.org/

Emergency Medical Technician (Chapter 26)

Bureau of Labor Statistics, U.S. Department of Labor, Occupational Outlook Handbook: EMTs and Paramedics. https://www.bls.gov/ooh/healthcare/emts-and-paramedics.htm September 2019

School CPR Free Student CPR by Protrainings.com https://schoolcpr.com/about/states-where-cpr-training-is-mandatory-for-high-school-graduation/

EMT and Paramedics Job Outlook Published April 12, 2019 https://www.bls.gov/ooh/healthcare/emts-and-paramedics.htm#tab-6

Pharmaceutical Sales Representative (Chapter 27)

Bureau of Labor Statistics, U.S. Department of Labor, Occupational Outlook Handbook: Wholesale and Manufacturing Sales Representatives. https://www.bls.gov/ooh/sales/wholesale-and-manufacturing-sales-representatives.htm September 2019

Mukherjee S. There's a Massive Pay Gap Between Pharma and Biotech Sales Reps Published June 23, 2016 http://fortune.com/2016/06/23/medical-sales-reps-pay-gap/

Pharmaceutical Research and Manufacturers of America guidelines for interaction with healthcare providers. Published February 2, 2017 http://www.phrma.org/codes-and-guidelines/code-on-interactions-with-health-care-professionals

S.301 - Physician Payments Sunshine Act of 2009 Published January 22, 2009 https://www.congress.gov/bill/111th-congress/senate-bill/301/text

Rath T. Strengths Finder 2.0. Published 2017 http://strengths.gallup.com/110440/About-StrengthsFinder-20.aspx

Top Medical Sales Companies to Work For — Best of 2019. Published 2019 https://www.medreps.com/medical-sales-careers/best-places-to-work/

The National Association of Pharmaceutical Representatives Published 2018 http://www.napsronline.org

Medical Writer (Chapter 28)

University of Chicago Graham School of Continuing Liberal and Professional Studies https://grahamschool.uchicago.edu/academic-programs/professional-development/medical-writing-and-editing

University of the Sciences https://www.usciences.edu/misher-college-of-arts-and-sciences/biomedical-writing-ms-certificates

Medical Writer Certified Credential

https://www.amwa.org/general/custom.asp?page=MWC

Glossary

ADC automated dispensing cabinet. An automated dispensing cabinet is a computerized drug storage cabinet or device designed mostly for use in hospitals. ADCs allow medications to be stored and dispensed near the point of care while controlling and tracking drug distribution.

adherence An active choice and describes the extent to which patients follow through with the prescribed treatment plan (e.g., medications, exercise, diet) while taking responsibility for their own health.

ADME Absorption, distribution, metabolism and excretion is how a medication distributes or moves within the body.

adverse drug reaction or drug reaction When a medication causes a problem or if the body responds badly to a medication. It is an unwanted occurrence that results from taking a medication correctly. The event is not expected by either the doctor or the patient and the effects can be reduced by lowering the dose or just stopping the medication altogether. An allergic reaction to a drug is one type of adverse drug reaction.

AIDS Acquired Immunodeficiency Syndrome. An infectious syndrome (or symptoms) caused by the human immunodeficiency virus (HIV) whereby the immune system is too weak to fight off infection. The HIV virus or AIDS used to be a death sentence because there were no treatments. There are now *many* treatments and it is a chronic infectious disease.

ALS (Advanced Life Support) Healthcare providers who oversee or manage cardiovascular emergencies are typically the medical professionals who receive ALS certification. Emergency response or emergency medicine professionals may obtain such training as well as workers in intensive and critical care units. ALS includes clinical protocols for urgently treating cardiac arrest, stroke, heart attack and other life-threatening cardiovascular emergencies.

anatomy The science associated with the structure of the body of humans, animals or other living organisms. Also, the study of the internal workings of the body or other things.

angioplasty (coronary angioplasty also known as percutaneous coronary intervention [PCI]) This is a procedure that restores blood flow to the coronary (heart) arteries when they become clogged. A doctor, usually an interventional radiologist, threads a thin tube (catheter) through a blood vessel in the arm or groin up to the involved site in the artery. The tube has a tiny balloon on the end. It is inflated to restore the flow. Angioplasty can improve symptoms such as chest pain or shortness of breath and doctors or other trained medical professionals can use it during a heart attack to quickly open a blocked artery and reduce the amount of heart damage.

AHA American Heart Association.

ARRT American Registry of Radiologic Technologists. This is the largest organization in the world that registers and awards 13 different credentials to radiologic technologists.

ASD Atrial Septal Defect, a hole in the wall between the two upper chambers of your heart (atria). The condition is present at birth (congenital).

ATR-BC Registered Art Therapist-Board Certified. This is the highest credential an Art Therapist can receive and is an assurance to employers, clients and the public that the therapist has met rigorous standards.

AVPT Austin Vocal Psychotherapist.

bariatrics The branch of medicine that deals with the causes, prevention, and treatment of obesity.

BCGP Board Certified in Geriatric Pharmacy. Geriatric Pharmacy Practice specializes in applying the knowledge of how drugs metabolize and work in older adults' bodies to optimize therapeutic outcomes. Currently there are more than 4,600 Board Certified Geriatric Pharmacists (BCGPs) in the United States.

BHSA Bachelor of Health Service Administration. This bachelor's degree course of study approaches healthcare delivery from a business and management perspective rather than a strictly medical standpoint.

bias A preconceived (an idea or opinion formed before having the actual evidence) opinion in favor of or against one thing, person or group compared with another, usually in a way that is unfair.

biologic pharmaceuticals/drugs Pharmaceuticals/drugs that are made using living organisms or parts of living organisms.

biotechnology Using living organisms or parts of living organisms to develop or make products (e.g., drugs, vaccines).

BLS (Basic Life Support) This usually refers to anyone who needs to know the basic principles of CPR, automated external defibrillator (AED) and other primary methods of lifesaving skills. Individuals, often who are not healthcare professionals, usually perform BLS. The more advanced level of training is referred to ACLS, Advanced Cardiac Life Support. ACLS is designed specifically for healthcare professionals and includes clinical protocols for urgently treating cardiac arrest, stroke, heart attack and other life-threatening cardiovascular emergencies.

board certification The process that a professional, including medical professionals, shows they have mastered basic knowledge and skills through written, practicing or simulation-based testing in a particular "practice" area.

BS - Bachelor of Science degree.

case management A collaborative process of assessment, planning, facilitation, care coordination, evaluation and advocacy for options and services to meet an individual's and family's comprehensive health needs through communication and available resources to promote quality, cost-effective outcomes.

cardiac ablation This is a procedure that scars a small area of the heart that may be causing an abnormal heart rhythm. Ablation can prevent the abnormal electrical signals or rhythms from moving through the heart and causing more problems.

cardiac biopsy (heart biopsy or myocardial biopsy) This is a procedure to detect heart disease. A small catheter with a grasping device on the end known as a bioptome is used to obtain a small piece of heart muscle tissue that is sent to a laboratory for analysis.

CBCN Certified Breast Cancer Nurse. CBCN is the only nationally accredited breast care nursing certification that is available exclusively to registered nurses. It encompasses the entire spectrum of breast care nursing practice.

CCC-SLP - Certificate of Clinical Competence in Speech Language Pathology. This is a nationally recognized professional credential that represents a level of excellence in the field of Speech Language Pathology.

CCM Certified Case Manager.

CDN Certified Dietician/Nutritionist. Some states have licensure laws for nutritionists. These credentials indicate that the individual has met the state's education or experience requirements for licensure.

CNSC Certified Nutrition Support Clinician. A certification of the National Board of Nutrition Support Certification (NBNSC). If credentialed, the individual has demonstrated that he or she has attained the skills and knowledge necessary to provide quality nutrition support care. This credential is available to dietitians, as well as to physicians, pharmacists, physician assistants and nurses.

clinical Related to observing and treating actual patients (pre-clinical studies are in animals).

clinical pathway An evidence based tool used to manage a specific group of patients with a predictable clinical course to improve outcomes.

clinical research Healthcare science performed on humans that helps determine the safety and effectiveness (how well it works) of drugs, devices, diagnostic products and treatment regimens.

clinical rotations Seeing patients in different treatment "settings" along with an instructor or preceptor (a preceptor is usually a skilled practitioner or faculty member).

CLT Clinical Laboratory Specialist.

compliance (healthcare) Following rules, regulations and laws relating to healthcare practices.

continuing education (CE) A term that encompasses a broad list of post secondary learning activities and programs, usually within a particular field.

coronary arteries The coronary arteries are the arteries of the coronary circulation, which transport blood into and out of the cardiac muscle (which encases the heart). The coronary arteries are mostly composed of right and left sides which both have branches.

coronary stenting Usually performed during angioplasty, a stent or a small wire mesh tube may be placed into the coronary artery to keep it open. Stents are placed when the coronary artery has narrowed or closed. The stent will open the coronary artery and decrease its chance of narrowing or closing.

cost effective An assessment of determination of the most efficient and least expensive approaches to providing health care and preventative medicine services.

CPhT Certified Pharmacy Technician.

CRNA Certified Registered Nurse Anesthetists. One of four Advanced Practice Nursing Licenses in the United States. The other three are Nurse Practitioners (NP), Certified Nurse Midwives and Clinical Nurse Specialists.

CRRN Certified Rehabilitation Registered Nurse. The CRRN credential is for nurses who assist individuals with disabilities and chronic illness to restore, maintain and promote optimal health.

CRT Certified Radiologic Technologist Certificate.

cultures (microbiological) Microbiological culture/microbial culture is a method of multiplying microscopic (small, often invisible to the eye) organisms by letting them reproduce in medium (e.g., agar plates, plates with certain chemicals) under controlled laboratory conditions. The medical profession uses microbial cultures to determine the type of organism and how many are present in the tested sample.

DDS/DMD Doctor of Dental Surgery and Doctor of Medicine in Dentistry are the same degrees. Dentists with these designations have the same education. Different universities determine what degree is awarded.

DNP Doctor of Nursing Practice degree. In the United States, the DNP is one of two doctorate degrees in nursing, the other being the PhD.

DO Doctor of Osteopathy or Doctor of Osteopathic Medicine.

DPM Doctor of Podiatric Medicine. Also known as a podiatric physician or surgeon. These professionals are qualified by their education and training to diagnose and treat conditions affecting the foot, ankle and related leg structures.

DPT Doctor of Physical Therapy. Currently, most physical therapy programs offer a DPT degree.

drug Formulary See Formulary.

drug-drug interactions This occurs when two or more drugs react with each other. Drugs interaction may make the drug less effective, cause unexpected side effects or increase a particular drug's action.

drug interactions There are three categories of drug interactions: drug-drug interactions, drug-food/beverage interactions and drug-condition interactions. An example of a drug-food/beverage interaction is when alcohol is mixed with some drugs which may cause tiredness or slow reactions.

drug reaction or adverse drug reaction When a medication causes a problem or if the body responds badly to a medication. It is an unwanted occurrence that results from taking a medication correctly. The event is not expected by either the doctor or the patient and the effects can be reduced by lowering the dose or just stopping the medication altogether. An allergic reaction to a drug is one type of adverse drug reaction.

EMT - Emergency Medical Technician.

FASHP Fellow of the American Society of Health-System Pharmacists. ASHP recognizes fellows as those pharmacists who have excelled in pharmacy practice and distinguished themselves through service and contributions to ASHP.

Food and Drug Administration (FDA) A federal agency of the United States Department of Health and Human services that is responsible for protecting and promoting public health through supervision and control of food safety, tobacco products, dietary supplements, vaccines, biopharmaceuticals, medical devices, animal food/feed, veterinary products and prescription and over-the-counter drugs.

formulary (or drug formulary) A list of drug products available for use within a particular hospital or (health) insurance plan. Not all drugs are included on the formulary.

entry level As it pertains to jobs, it is normally designed for recent graduates of a given field and typically does not require prior work experience in that particular field.

evidence Using available proven valid facts or information.

evidence-based medicine Making decisions related to health or providing care by using the best available evidence with practice experience and other resources.

formulary An official list of drugs available or covered within a particular health-system (e.g., hospital, managed care plan) or insurance.

gerontological Relating to the aging population or geriatric patients.

hematocrit The volume of packed red blood cells in a blood specimen.

hemoglobin The oxygen-carrying part of a red blood cell.

hospice A home providing care for the sick or terminally ill. It is also for patients whose condition is such that a doctor would not be surprised if the patient died within the next six months. This does not mean the patient is going to die in the next six months--it simply means that he or she has a condition that makes dying a realistic possibility.

hospital protocols Official procedure or system of rules in how to proceed within a particular hospital.

infused pharmaceuticals/drugs Drugs that are received intravenously (in a vein) over a period of time (usually at least 15 minutes).

institutional Occurring in a hospital, or other "building".

L-CAT Licensed Creative Arts Therapist (music, dance/movement, art, drama, poetry).

LCSW - R Licensed Clinical Social Worker - R designation in New York State allows Psychotherapy Privilege. Psychotherapy in the content of LCSW practice uses verbal methods in interpersonal relationships with the intent of assisting patients to modify attitudes and behavior which are intellectually, socially or emotionally maladaptive.

LMHC Licensed Mental Health Counselor.

MA - Master of Arts degree.

managed care - A system in healthcare where patients agree to visit only certain doctors and hospitals. A managing company monitors treatment costs.

market share The part of a market controlled by a specific company or product.

MDS - Master of Dental Surgery. A postgraduate dental course that takes from two to three years to complete.

medical intern The first year of medical training for doctors following graduation from medical school.

medical resident The second year (and possibly additional years) of medical training for doctors following their internship (starting two years following graduation from medical school).

medical team A group of healthcare workers usually including a physician, who are responsible for patients' medical needs while they are in the hospital. "Team approach" is now the most common form of patient management in the United States.

Medication Therapy Management See MTM.

medication reconciliation This is the process of creating the most accurate possible list of all patients' medications. This includes the drug name, dosage, frequency and route. These are compared against the physician's admission, transfer and/or discharge orders. The goal is to provide the correct list. It sounds basic, but it very important and often not correct, since there are so many different variables.

mental health A person's psychological (related to the mind) and emotional well-being.

MRI Magnetic Resonance Imaging. This test uses very strong magnets, radio waves and a computer to make detailed pictures inside the body. The medical team can use this test to diagnose illness or see how a patient has responded to a treatment.

MPAS Master of Physician Assistant Studies.

MS Master of Science degree.

MT-BC Music Therapist-Board Certified.

MTM Medication Therapy Management. MTM practitioners are usually pharmacists. Working as an MTM pharmacist requires more than assessing medications for specific use, effectiveness, safety and adherence issues. It also requires patient counseling that factors in patients' emotional, financial and cultural states.

Multidisciplinary Combining several specialized branches of learning or fields of expertise. An example is a group of healthcare providers including a nurse, pharmacist, social worker, physician, dietician, PA and NP.

NP Nurse Practitioner. One of four Advanced Practice Nursing Licenses in the United States. The other three are Certified Registered Nurse Anesthetists (CRNA), Certified Nurse Midwives and Clinical Nurse Specialists.

OCN Oncology Certified Nurse. To become an OCN you must have a BSN, have worked as an RN for at least one year and have completed at least 1,000 hours working in Clinical Oncology.

on call Availability on short notice. In the medical field, usually physicians are "on call" meaning that they are at the hospital, ready to work at moment's notice.

oncology Of or pertaining to the prevention, diagnosis and treatment of cancer.

OTR/L Occupational Therapist Registered/ Licensed.

outcomes End results of treatments or interventions (the goal of care is to have positive outcomes).

P & T Committee (see Pharmacy and Therapeutics Committee)

PA Physician Assistant.

PA-C Certified Physician Assistant. The National Commission of Certification certifies these PAs. This certification requires 100 hours of continuing medical education every two years, along with passing a national recertification exam every six years to maintain this certification.

PBM Pharmacy Benefit Managers. A PBM is a third-party administrator (or company) that manages and delivers prescription drug benefits for individuals who are part of a group or plan. Different pharmacy plans include: commercial health plans (e.g., large employer groups like Verizon® or Xerox®), self-insured employer plans (small business), Medicare Part D plans (drug benefits for elderly patients), federal employees (e.g., the US government) and state government employee plans (e.g., New York, Florida, Kentucky, Maine). Their goal is to reduce prescription drug costs and improve convenience and safety for individuals within the drug plans they cover.

PCR Polymerase Chain Reaction is a laboratory technique that makes multiple copies of a DNA segment. It is very precise and medical professionals use it to enlarge or copy a specific DNA target from a mixture of DNA molecules. It has become an indispensable tool in research and diagnostic medicine.

pharmaceutical company A drug sponsor, marketer and/or manufacturer of drugs.

pharmaceutical industry Pertains to all drug sponsors, marketers and/or manufacturers.

pharmacokinetics The study of drug movement through the body, including processes of absorption, distribution, localization in tissues, biotransformation and excretion.

pharmacology The science that deals with the origin, nature, chemistry, effects and uses of drugs.

pharmacotherapy Medical treatment using drugs.

pharmacovigilance The pharmacological science relating to the collection, detection, assessment, monitoring, and prevention of adverse effects with pharmaceutical products.

Pharmacy and Therapeutics Committee (P & T Committee) This committee is composed of actively participating physicians, other prescribers, pharmacists, nurses, administrators, quality-improvement managers, and other healthcare professionals and staff who participate in the medication-use process in a particular health-system. All health-systems have a P & T Committee. The committee serves in an evaluative, educational and advisory capacity to the medical staff and organization, for all matters relating to medication use. The overarching purposes of the P&T committee are drug policy development, communication and education and formulary management. The P & T Committee also takes actions to prevent, monitor and evaluate adverse drug reactions and medication errors in the healthcare settings.

pharmacy fellowship This is a post-graduate program (after obtaining a PharmD) that focuses on developing skills to make a pharmacist successful, typically, in the pharmaceutical industry. A few fellowships are not in the pharmaceutical industry, but the majority are geared towards this type of practice. These fellowship programs can be between one to two years in length. These fellows gain experience in various departments within a pharmaceutical company such as drug information, health economics and pharmacovigilance. These programs are highly competitive and usually prepare the individual for work in research. There are also fellowships in academia, which prepares the pharmacist for a career in teaching at an academic institution.

pharmacy residency This is a post-graduate program (after obtaining a PharmD) focused on clinical pharmacy practice in an institutional (mostly hospital) setting. These are typically broken into Post-graduate year 1 (PGY1) and Post-graduate year 2 (PGY2). Residents who successfully complete a PGY1 would have to apply for a PGY2 program. Completing a PGY2 is not mandatory after completing a PGY1 program. The PGY2 year is usually more specialized than the first year.

PharmD Doctor of Pharmacy. Currently, the most common entry level pharmacy degree awarded in the United States.

PhD Doctor of Philosophy. In the United States, the PhD is one of two doctorate degrees in nursing, the other is the DNP.

physiology The science that deals with the functions of living organisms and its parts, and of the physical and chemical factors involved.

preceptor An experiential educator. A preceptor is a pharmacy practitioner who, by acting as a role model where they practice pharmacy, helps students acquire the abilities (knowledge, skills and attitudes) necessary for providing patient-centered pharmaceutical care.

primary care Care provided by physicians specifically trained for and skilled in overall "first contact" and continuing care for persons with any undiagnosed sign, symptom or health concern.

prophylaxis Action taken to prevent disease, especially by specified means or against a specified disease.

psychotherapy The treatment of mental disorders by psychological therapy rather than by medical therapy (e.g., drugs).

PT Physical Therapist.

pull-through strategy A business tactic that creates interest for a specific product or service within a target audience and then demands the product. This causes the product to "pull" through the manufacturer's sales channel to the product partners.

push-through strategy A business tactic that moves products and services through channel partners to the consumer. A push strategy uses marketing channels, such as trade promotions, to "push" a product or service through to the sales channel.

quality control A system for proving and preserving a desired quality level in a product or process by careful planning, use of proper equipment, continued inspection and corrective action as needed.

RD Registered Dietician.

RDH Registered Dental Hygienist.

regulations An authoritative rule issued by a governing agency.

RN Registered Nurse.

RN-BC Board Certified Nurse. Anyone with this credential after his or her name means that he or she is a registered nurse who has achieved board certification in his or her specialty. The professional nursing practice may involve patient care or another aspect of nursing.

shadowing Observing someone doing his or her job. In shadowing one has the opportunity to see someone actually in a job that is of interest to them. In addition, because one is at an actual site, one can see inside the workplace.

side effects An undesired effect that occurs when the medication is administered regardless of the dose. Unlike adverse events, side effects are usually predicted by the physician and the patient is counseled to be aware of the effects that could happen while on therapy. Side effects can resolve on their own with time after taking the medication for several weeks. An example of a side effect would be using a diabetes drug that causes weight loss in obese diabetic patients, due to its potential weight loss benefit.

specialty A particular area or branch of medical science to which one devotes their professional attention.

specialty pharmaceuticals Also known as specialty drugs, these are a fairy recent designation of drugs that are classified as high cost, high complexity and/or high touch. Specialty drugs are often biologic drugs that are injectable or infused. However, some may be oral medications. The medical profession uses some oral specialty drugs to treat ailments such as cancer, multiple sclerosis, rheumatoid arthritis and psoriasis.

specialty pharmacy The service created to mange the handling and special requirements of specialty pharmaceuticals/ drugs, including storage, dispensing, distribution, reimbursement, case management and other patient specific services for those with rare and/or chronic

diseases requiring these medications.

specimens A sample of something, such as tissue, cells or blood that is taken for medical testing.

Standard Operating Procedures (SOPs) A set of step-by-step instructions that an organization compiles to help workers carry out operations. The purpose of SOPs is to achieve efficiency, quality output and uniform performance, while decreasing miscommunication and failure to comply with industry regulations.

STEM Science, Technology, Engineering and Math.

sterile field An area free of microorganisms. Usually it is an area immediately around a patient that has been prepared for a surgical procedure. The sterile field includes the scrubbed team members, properly attired and all furniture and fixtures in the area.

Territory Region. In the example of a pharmaceutical sales representative's territory, this is the area where he or she can find "clients". It can include a city, a state and/or a number of states. The representative's "clients" could include physician's offices, hospitals, managed care plans, PBMs and pharmacies.

toxicology The branch of science concerned with the nature, effects and detection of chemicals and poisonous substances on people, animals and the environment. It includes measuring and analyzing potential toxins, intoxicating or banned substances and prescription medications present. If it is in a person's body, then it is clinical toxicology.

Transitions of Care (TOC) This refers to patients' movement between healthcare practitioners, settings, areas within a hospital/health-system and home, as their condition and care needs change. Hospitals must improve the effectiveness of transitions of care to reduce both hospital readmission rates and adverse events.

vital signs Clinical measurements specifically pulse rate, temperature, respiration rate and blood pressure. These all indicate the state of a patient's essential body functions.

webinars A seminar or talk conducted over the internet.

Index